The Western Way of Death

Malcolm Carruthers, M.D.

The Western Way of Death

Stress, Tension and Heart Attacks

PANTHEON BOOKS
A Division of Random House, New York

First American Edition

Copyright © 1974 by Malcolm Carruthers
All rights reserved under International and Pan-American
Copyright Conventions. Published in the United States by
Pantheon Books, a division of Random House, Inc., New
York. Originally published in Great Britain by Davis-
Poynter Ltd., London.

Library of Congress Cataloging in Publication Data

Carruthers, Malcolm, 1938-
    The Western Way of Death: Stress, Tension, and Heart
Attacks.

    Bibliography: p. 135
    1. Stress (Physiology)   2. Heart failure.
3. Death—Causes.   I. Title.
QP82.2.S8C37 1974   616.1'2   73-18714
ISBN 0-394-49160-2

Manufactured in the United States of America

The author wishes to thank Pergamon Press Ltd
for permission to quote the list on pages 73–74
from Dr R. H. Rahe's "Social Stress and Illness
Onset," *Journal of Psychosomatic Research*, Vol.
8, 1964.

For Janet

Contents

Acknowledgements

My thanks are above all due to Dr Taggart who first stimulated my interest in this field, and with whom practically all the clinical work has been done. Without him this work would never have been begun, let alone completed.

At the Middlesex Hospital, Professor R. H. S. Thompson helped to initiate this project, and Dr Walter Somerville has given continued guidance and encouragement throughout.

In its continuation at the Institute of Ophthalmology, Professor Norman Ashton has been unfailingly helpful in prompting and advising on this work. A generous grant for Auto-Analyser equipment by the Medical Research Council made the many analyses involved in these studies possible.

I would also like to express my thanks to Miss Eileen Willmott, Mr W. Hiley, Mr Brian Augier and other members of the staff at the Institute of Ophthalmology for technical help. In addition, I am grateful to Cynthia Read for the immense amount of patient work carried out in the preparation of the manuscript, and to my father, G. H. Carruthers, for preparing the index.

In the racing-driver studies, my thanks are due to Dr Tony Goodwin who, in addition to being a subject on five separate occasions, assisted with the organization at the circuits; all the drivers taking part; Motor Racing Stables Ltd, British Racing and Sports Car Club, British Automobile Club, and the officials at Continental circuits, including Nurburgring, Spa and Mugello, also David Gibbons for a large amount of help with the electro-cardiographic techniques involved. The work was supported by grants from the Medical Commission on Accident Prevention, the Automobile Association and C.I.B.A. Ltd. In studies on public speaking and swimming, considerable help in organization and the finding of volunteers was provided by Mrs Sheila Harrison of the British Heart Foundation.

The studies on television watchers were only made possible by the kind assistance of Dr Effron Gwynne-Jones of the Further Education Department of the B.B.C. Thanks are also due to members of the Audio-Visual Department of Moorfields Eye Hospital. C.I.B.A. provided both financial assistance and some of the volunteers for the studies on film viewing.

For the study of athletics, my thanks are due to Mr Frank Dick of the Scottish Amateur Athletic Joint Coaching Committee.

The investigations on physical stress in unfit individuals were initiated by the late Dr Harold Lewis, and continued within the framework of the Exercise therapy study, supported by the Medical Research Council under the direction of Dr Otto Edholm. This work was carried out at the City Gymnasium with the help of healthy volunteers and patients of Dr Peter Nixon attending for cardiac rehabilitation. The incentive and thought behind these studies is almost entirely due to Dr Nixon and Alistair Murray, who designed the exercise schedules involved as well as supervizing their application.

Last, but far from least, I would like to thank my wife, Dr Janet Carruthers, for her tolerance of the stresses involved.

Introduction

It is an ironic fact that while half the world's population is dying as a result of diseases of poverty (largely starvation and infection), the other half is succumbing to diseases of affluence. Foremost among the latter are traffic accidents, lung cancer and, above all, coronary thrombosis. This last disease alone caused about 200,000 deaths in Great Britain last year, and regularly achieves a 'megadeath' in North America.

The remedies of affluence, although effective against the diseases of poverty, are curiously inadequate in combating diseases of affluence. For example, although safer cars and better surgery may increase the proportion of people surviving road accidents, a steady increase in the number of vehicles ensures the progress of this fashionable way of death. Detailed and statistically elegant comparisons of survival times of people with cancer of the lung have, except in the rare case which is diagnosed early, failed to demonstrate any appreciable difference between treatment with surgery, radiotherapy, drugs or fresh air. Indeed, Sir Francis Chichester might have put up a good argument for the latter. Prevention, however, by alteration of smoking habits and, in some fortunate areas by the lessening of atmospheric pollution, is causing a levelling off of the mortality from this condition.

Unfortunately the same cannot be said for coronary heart disease, which has become by far the biggest single peacetime killer of Western man. In spite of all the 'wonders' of modern medicine, it has also resulted in an actual reduction in the life expectancy of the adult American male, who has been quoted as being currently more concerned with the state of his coronary arteries than with thoughts of the number of inter-continental ballistic missiles pointing at him. This is understandable as it probably was not a rocket that got his boss last week. It cannot even be claimed that it is lack of an early warning system that defeats attempts to prevent coronary artery disease. The changes in blood chemistry and in walls of the arteries occur over several years and warning symptoms and signs usually build up for some months before the heart attack. Lack of knowledge of the root causes, and hence of the appropriate remedies to halt, or even reverse, the inward arterial rot defeats preventive measures.

It is for these reasons that a book such as this has been written. No attempt is made to cover with over-all even emphasis the network of detailed, complex, and often contradictory evidence that surrounds the subject of coronary artery disease. The aim is to produce a light-hearted account of just one of many theories currently being investigated in this field.

The theory is that the combination of a high level of emotional activity, together with a low level of physical activity, deranges body chemistry and is the major cause of heart disease. This personal view claims to be in accordance with the majority of observable facts and presents a chain of events, each link of which can and must be tested. By forming a clearly-defined picture out of the jig-saw pieces of information available, it is hoped to offer those who find the basic idea sufficiently convincing some guide-lines in taking appropriate evasive action. At least if other more important and as yet undiscovered causes of coronary heart disease are suddenly revealed, the only side-effects of this book will be to assist the few people who manage to lessen their rage reactions both in and out of cars together with a minute reduction in the consumption of cigarettes. As in the rest of medicine the aim is 'firstly to do no harm'.

1. Emotion as a cause of heart attacks

The Heart Attack

Let's begin by getting clear what we mean by a heart attack. It is when the blood supply to the heart of an adult becomes inadequate in either quantity or quality. Although the underlying condition develops slowly, the final attack is usually dramatically rapid in onset, and is surrounded by one or other of a combination of four events of increasing order of severity:

1 Angina

A tight, crushing or pressing pain in the chest, sometimes going into the arms or neck. This has been most vividly described by those experiencing it as being like a heavy weight on the chest. It is thought to be partly due to the heart muscle going short of oxygen, and partly due to its being stretched by blood accumulating inside the heart.

2 Breathlessness

This is caused by blood not being adequately pumped

through the lungs, and also fluid accumulating in them, thus giving a form of internal drowning.

3 Loss of consciousness

The blood supply to the brain is reduced, and like the other but less essential organs, without adequate circulation it stops working. As it is the most active tissue in the body, it is also the first to fail. If the heart should stop beating completely, consciousness is lost within a minute, and after three minutes without circulation the brain is effectively dead. Without oxygen not only is the machine stopped but the machinery is wrecked. By comparison, the heart can survive without oxygen for half an hour, and other muscles and the kidneys for an hour. This is why it is the speed of starting external heart massage and mouth-to-mouth breathing, rather than the elegance of the technique used, which is important in treating an unconscious heart attack victim.

4 Death

Nearly half of the early deaths from heart attack occur within the first hour. Early deaths usually result from the heart beating irregularly for a while, and then just stopping. With variable degrees of success this can be treated by thumping the chest wall over the heart or, in some ambulances and hospitals, by giving the heart a short sharp electric shock. Even when the heart has re-started recovery is not guaranteed, as it may beat for a while and then stop again.

Later deaths are caused by a wide variety of complications. These include gradual increase or recurrence of the early troubles and progressive weakening and softening of the area of the heart muscle affected. This may even burst, so that the person dies literally of a broken heart.

Depressing as this picture is, seventy per cent of people survive their first heart attack and return to their previous way of life, albeit with a few extra pills and muttered warnings about 'taking it easy' from their medical advisors. Conventional present-day long-term treatment of a heart attack is as vague as knowledge of its causes, so it is worth taking a look at the way in which the various theories have grown up.

The Fall and Rise of the Emotional Theory

Ancient Egyptian medicine was mainly concerned with driving out evil spirits by a series of empirical remedies to be found in the thirty-two Hermetic books of the god Thoth, teacher of Alchemy. As long as the physician followed the exact treatment specified in these books to the hieroglyphic, no one thought any the worse of him if the patient died. Traces of this hermetic sealing of the mind can be found in some of the ineffective but orthodox treatments applied to heart disease today. The heart was considered to be the most important organ in the body, and was the only one left in place during embalming. Since during life remedies were applied to overcome possession by devils, any medicine taken had to be directed to the scene of action by incantations such as one in the Ebers Papyrus dated about 500 BC: 'Welcome, remedy! Welcome! that dost drive away that which is in this my heart and in these my limbs'. Such positive psychotherapy is sadly lacking in most drug prescriptions and may account for the popularity of some health foods which have similar inspiring messages on the label. Even animal fats, which are now under a dietetic cloud, were looked upon as being especially beneficial to health.

Probably the earliest recorded heart attack is described in the Old Testament dating from about 1050 BC. The victim was a very rich and important man called Nabal who was renowned for being 'churlish and evil in his doings' (*Samuel*, Book I, Chapter 25). No one could speak to him without him losing his temper, and he finally made the nearly fatal mistake of insulting King David. When Nabal heard that it was only his wife's intercession that had prevented David from killing him, his remorse appears to have been such that 'his heart died within him'. This story suggests that from earliest times it has been thought that the emotion of anger, particularly when directed against oneself, could damage the heart.

The early Greeks, beginning with Aesculapius, from about 1000 BC began to transform medicine from a mystical art to an objective science. In the temples of health which were set up to honour this god, the patient had to make a sacrificial offer on arrival and purify himself by bathing. He then underwent curative 'temple sleep' which is still to this day enforced in hospitals albeit by the rigorous administration of sleeping pills. Sleep therapy prolonged for up to a week, with the patient kept asleep by drugs for most of the period, has recently been found to be a very effective treatment immediately after a heart attack. Also physical therapy in the form of a healthy regime and exercise in pleasant surroundings to complete the cure, are now even more important in treating heart patients than when they were first applied to ill people in general 3,000 years ago.

Although the Greeks brought in the idea that the brain, and not the heart, was the organ which was most important to the senses, it was one of their physicians, Empedocles, who laid the foundation of the humoral theory of disease. He was convinced that the heart distributed the life-giving force *pneuma* to all parts of the body. To ensure that his theories survived, and in an abortive attempt to get promoted to a god, he finally leapt into the crater of Mount Etna. Hippocrates, however, did not allow his arguments to become so heated. He insisted on an ordered, scientific, and objective study of disease. Among his most important teachings was the idea that both the environment and the habits of the people living in it largely determined what types of disease would be common. This epidemological approach to disease is again rightly coming into prominence in the search for the underlying factors in the commonest cause of death in western communities, coronary artery disease.

Greek medicine was absorbed by the expanding Roman Empire and after a somewhat fallow period it was revived by Galen about AD 150. As well as being a brilliant clinician and experimenter, he is said to have produced over 500 books. Apart from their great number, the force and clarity of these works were such that they dominated medical thought and practice for the next 1,200 years. They became part of several religious doctrines so that to question them was heresy. This made for stability in medical practice, but not progress in medical research. Thought on both the function and diseases of the heart was thus effectively stifled for a millenium until the discovery by William Harvey that blood circulated round the body from the arteries to the veins under the action of the heart. The publication of this unorthodox theory in 1628 made its author very unpopular, especially as he gave step-by-step proof. In this book on the circulation of the blood he also gave the interesting case history of a 'strong man who, having received an injury and affront from one more powerful than himself, and upon whom he could not have his revenge, was so overcome with hatred and spite and passion, that at last he fell into a strange distemper, suffering from extreme oppression and pain of the heart and breast', from which the patient died within a few years.

The peak of the emotional theory of heart disease was reached around 1700 with the writings of the famous English surgeon John Hunter, who firmly believed that strong emotion could bring on a heart attack. His views were epitomized by the saying: 'My life is at the mercy of any fool who shall put me in a passion'. He proved his point by dying abruptly during a meeting of the board of governors of his hospital.

Why then, after 4,000 years, did views change on the cause of heart trouble? It is a classical example of the dubious triumph of science over common experience. Medicine entered an age of detailed study of structure, function and, as the sum of knowledge grew, specialization. This process began with elegant dissections and descriptions of the heart's own blood supply, the coronary arteries. Two in number, a right and a left, they get their name because they form a circle, or coronet, round the heart. They spring from the biggest blood vessel in the body, the aorta, just as it leaves the top of the heart and

17

is beginning to arch over, giving off branches to the head and arms, before doubling back to supply the rest of the body. Though the blood vessel from which they came is as thick as the average domestic water pipe, the coronary arteries are as thin as a drinking straw. This circle of arteries goes round the outside of the heart, branching progressively, to form a complete network which supplies blood to all parts of the heart. This forms, and indeed looks like, the roots of the arterial tree, clasping and nourishing that fountain of life, the heart. Soon after these arteries had been described, it was noticed that they, like many other arteries in the body, could be affected by a mysterious inward rot. This went in a series of easily recognizable stages which were therefore eagerly described and categorized by the anatomists of disease. The process begins insidiously with the gradual accumulation of yellow fatty material beneath the living membrane of both large arteries, especially the aorta, and smaller arteries such as the coronaries. The inside of the vessels then looks as though some invisible hand has gone along them plastering thick flecks of yellow paint on their walls. Over the months and years more and more fat gathers between the elastic and muscle tissue making up the arterial wall and its lining membrane. This fat forms round or oval bumps in the wall of the artery which are most marked where the arteries divide. The final stage of the process is when the smooth inner membrane breaks down over these collections of fat. The rough warty, porridgy, mess which is then exposed gives the condition its medical name, atheroma, from the Greek word for oats. The process can be likened in appearance to the gradual furring up of water pipes in a central heating system, except that it is much more patchy and irregular. Instead of flowing evenly over surfaces as smooth as a rifle barrel, the blood churns its turbulent way along the roughened, softened and narrowed channels inside the affected vessels.

All these changes can go on silently at various rates within the arteries supplying such vital organs as the heart, brain and kidneys. Either gradually or abruptly, the villain then shows his hand in the final act as complications, which directly affect the patient's health, set in. Most commonly a blood clot forms on the roughened wall of one of the arteries. In the heart this causes the true 'coronary thrombosis'. In spite of the widespread use of this term an actual blood clot blocking a large branch of one of the coronary arteries is only found in half the cases of 'heart attack', though a significant atheromatous change in these vessels is constantly present. In these no-blood-clot cases it seems likely that the heart suddenly needed more blood to meet a physical, or, more often, emotional emergency, and either the quantity or quality of the blood reaching it through the narrowed vessels proved inadequate.

Sometimes some of the warty excrescences on the roughened walls of the arteries affected by the atheromatous process break off. They are then swept off in the eddying current of blood to lodge as a plug in a smaller artery down-stream. The effects of the resulting blockage can be disastrous where ever it occurs in the body. Such stalactites of debris projecting from the arterial wall hang all too literally like the Sword of Damocles over the lives of people in whom atheromatous changes are far advanced. Though very fortunately a rare event, one of the large arteries affected by this softening may even begin to tear at these weak spots, usually with spectacular results.

Such then is the catalogue of calamities attributed to the gradual but progressive atheromatous changes seen in the walls of arteries by the earliest investigations of the anatomy of illness in the eighteenth and nineteenth centuries. After the dissectors, hot in pursuit of the ultimate truth, came the microscopists. Attention was diverted from the whole patient to elegantly thin slices of the wall of his blood vessels. As expected, each stage of the process showed more and more fat gathering beneath the lining of the artery, eventually bursting through it. More revealing was the fact that unmistakable crystals of the best-known fat in the body, cholesterol, were recognized in these sites and became the hallmarks of the condition

19

as long as one hundred years ago. There followed no major advance for about fifty years in knowledge of this condition. This pause in an era of otherwise rapid scientific advancement was due to a combination of factors. To begin with the condition used to be relatively uncommon, especially before the age of fifty, and was therefore regarded as an interesting example of the changes associated with ageing. Tuberculosis was still the captain of the men of death in the middle-aged, and this position was only usurped by heart disease after the Second World War. Since then the atheromatous changes described have been seen in arteries all over the body in a greater proportion of people at an earlier and earlier age. Indeed in men over the age of twenty, some degree of this change has become almost the norm. Of 3,000 American soldiers below the age of thirty killed in the Korean war, fifty per cent showed some changes and twenty-five per cent marked changes in their coronary arteries. Similarly, among 400 young men of the Royal Air Force dying in crashes, thirty per cent showed severe changes and forty-five per cent moderate changes, so that only twenty-five per cent were completely free. Such figures only slightly lessen the surprise of the British Heart Foundation's estimate that in Great Britain and North America half of the adult male deaths are due to coronary artery disease, and that the proportion is still increasing. Even when heart attacks started to become a fashionable way of death at an increasingly early age, progress in discovering their causes still lagged. This was partly because scientific theories naturally tend to be based on what has been most recently observed and can most easily be measured. Cholesterol was the ideal choice of culprit as it had been found on the scene of the crime by microscopists. Its foot-prints in the shape of characteristic clefts could be clearly seen in the walls of some affected arteries, where it could be stained a spectacular and guilt-ridden red colour. The chemists were also happy to testify to cholesterol being the 'bad egg'. There was plenty of it to measure, both in the blood and in the food, and the levels of the two and heart disease tended to bear a suspicious, albeit inconstant relationship. Being nice and stable both in and out of the body, and not one of these will-o'-the-wisp compounds whose blood levels vary wildly during the day and disappear as soon as you think you've got them trapped in a test tube, it was a sitting duck for the collection of chemically incriminating evidence. From here it was a brief exercise in *ad hoc* reasoning to the 'It's what you eat that does it' school of thought that holds sway to this day. This originally suggested that a high cholesterol diet raises blood cholesterol to a level where it is gradually deposited in the walls of the blood vessels and builds up to cause atheroma. For various reasons, this theory was later broadened to include saturated animal fat among the dietary 'baddies' in the dock with cholesterol. Unsaturated vegetable fats, especially the polyunsaturated ones, were cast in the role of 'goodies' who were able to combat the evil effects of the 'baddies'. The market soon became saturated with unsaturated food products. This was good for the circulation of grocery products and magazines with complicated diet sheets, but appeared to have little effect on the coronary circulation. Heart attack rates obstinately continued to rise.

Specialization within medicine probably has to bear some of the blame for the slow advance in knowledge of the causes of heart trouble. Pathologists could describe what happened but not why it happened. Blood chemists could measure rises in blood fats but not explain them. Cardiologists could diagnose heart trouble and save some patients during the acute attack, but not prevent them. Heart surgeons could even plumb in a completely new heart, which in some cases then underwent the same arterial changes as the old one.

The revival of the theory that emotional stress might be a major cause of heart disease was therefore left to general physicians and general practitioners. The latter especially saw evidence in their everyday experience of viewing people's illness against the background of home and work that there was a characteristic pattern of life preceding many of the deaths from heart disease. This could be characterized as an irregular, self-destructive way of life, primarily dominated by emotions of aggression, anger and ambition. These are inevitably accompanied by secondary problems arising from booze, birds, a bulging bread-basket, burning the candle at both ends, and blood pressure. The coronary-prone pattern of behaviour was classified on a more serious psychological basis by two very eminent workers in America, Rosenman and Friedman, who have studied a large group of men in San Francisco. They divided this population into two groups according to their individual characteristics. Type A behaviour subjects were defined as those showing great competitiveness, rapidity of thought and action, together with time and deadline consciousness. Type B behaviour pattern was the reverse, being not competitive, easy going and slower, but often no less effective in the long run. When these two groups, living in the same community, eating the same food and smoking roughly similar amounts were compared, it was found that the Group A individuals suffered more than six times as many heart attacks as the Group B personalities. Also the Group A who died for any reason showed six times as much coronary artery disease, and before death had higher levels of cholesterol and other blood fats likely to lead up to this condition. An additional important factor in the renaissance of the idea of emotion underlying heart disease was that it became possible to measure emotion in terms of the hormones adrenaline and its parent compound noradrenaline released under nervous stimulation. The result of this combination of direct studies in the field, and chemical studies in the laboratory was the theory that forms the theme of this book.

Emotion as a Cause of Heart Disease

Man has not changed significantly in either bodily or chemical form since the process of civilization began. To be effective as a 'weapon-toting wolf' as Desmond Morris has so vividly described him, primitive man possessed a set of automatically aroused chemical alarm reactions. These reactions immediately prepared his body for active

IMPORTANT QUESTIONS & ANSWERS ABOUT THE CHAMPUS SUPPLEMENT

Q. Who is eligible to apply?

A. All U.S.A. members under age 65 who are entitled to retired, retainer, or equivalent pay, spouses under age 65 of active duty or retired members, and their unmarried, dependent children from birth to age 21 or to age 23 if a full-time student are eligible to apply. Unmarried widows or widowers and children of deceased active duty or deceased retirees are also eligible for coverage.

Q. When will my coverage become effective?

A. Your insurance coverage will become effective on the first day of the calendar month coincident with or next following receipt of your application and first premium payment.

Q. What is my proof of coverage?

A. An individual certificate of insurance will be sent to you, stating the essential features of coverage and to whom benefits are payable. Complete instruction for filing a claim will also be included.

Q. Can the insurance company cancel my coverage?

A. Under the U.S.A. CHAMPUS Supplement Plan, your coverage remains in effect until age 65 as long as you pay your premiums on time, remain a member of U.S.A., and the master contract remains in force. Your dependents' coverage will remain in effect until your coverage terminates, or until they cease to be eligible for coverage.

Q. What are pre-existing conditions?

A. Pre-existing conditions are those injuries sustained or conditions for which you received medical treatment or advice from a physician within 12 months prior to the effective date of your coverage. Such conditions will not be covered until after a period of 12 consecutive months has elapsed, during which no medical treatment or advice is received, or you have been covered for 24 consecutive months, whichever occurs earlier.

Q. HOW DO I APPLY?

A. 1. Complete the application on the reverse side, sign, and date where indicated.

2. Determine your premium amount and make your check for the first month's premium and membership fee, if not already a member, payable to U.S.A.

3. Mail your completed application and check to:

   U.S.A.
   8027 Leesburg Pike
   Suite 710
   Vienna, Virginia 22180

This brochure provides a brief description of the benefits available. Complete details may be found in master policy 7432 underwritten by North American Life and Casualty Company, Minneapolis, Minnesota 55403

Advertising Supplement to the Army, Navy, Air Force Times

CHAMPUS Supplement Enrollment Form

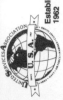

Established 1962

I hereby apply for enrollment in the CHAMPUS Supplement Plan, as provided for in the Group Master Policy **#7432** issued to U.S.A. by the North American Life and Casualty Co. I understand that my insurance coverage will be effective on the first day of the calendar month coincident with or next following receipt of my application and the first premium payment.

1. Member's Name

   Last _____ First _____ MI ___

2. Address _____

   City _____ State _____ Zip _____

3. Branch of service _____

4. Member's date of birth _____

5. Coverage desired *(Please check)*.

   Retired Member
   ☐ Inpatient only
   ☐ In- and Outpatient

   Spouse of Active Member
   ☐ Inpatient only
   ☐ In- and Outpatient

   Spouse of Retired Member
   ☐ Inpatient only
   ☐ In- and Outpatient

   Each Child of Active Member
   ☐ Inpatient only
   ☐ In- and Outpatient

   Each Child of Retired Member
   ☐ Inpatient only
   ☐ In- and Outpatient

   ☐ I am enclosing my $5.00 Lifetime Membership Fee
   ☐ I am a member of U.S.A.

6. Complete for each dependent for whom coverage is desired:

   Spouse   Last Name _____ First _____ MI ___ Birthdate _____

   Children Last Name _____ First _____ MI ___ Birthdate _____

   Last Name _____ First _____ MI ___ Birthdate _____

   Last Name _____ First _____ MI ___ Birthdate _____

   If additional names, attach separate sheet of paper.

   NOTICE: The following question must be answered: Do you understand that this program does not cover conditions for which the above persons to be covered have received medical treatment or advice within 12 months prior to the date individual coverage goes into effect, but these conditions will be covered after any covered person has received no treatment or advice for 12 consecutive months after the individual effective date or after a period of 24 consecutive months insured, regardless of treatment, whichever is less?

   YES _____ NO _____

7. _____

   Member's Signature   Date

   MAKE CHECK PAYABLE TO U.S.A. and mail to:
   United Services Association 8027 Leesburg Pike—Suite 710 Vienna, Virginia 22180

physical hand-to-hand fighting or, if the threat was too great, for fleeing. To understand how these alarm reactions may have become inappropriate to modern man we must consider their basic chemistry. When someone is emotionally aroused by anger, fear or excitement of almost any kind, the part of the brain most concerned with automatic responses, the mid-brain, is activated. This 'emergency control' centre has lines of communication with all the organs in the body. These make up the sympathetic (*sym* – with, *pathos* – feeling) nervous system of the body. The effects of its action can be most clearly seen in someone who has had a fright. Their paleness is due to contraction and narrowing of the blood vessels in the skin. This makes more blood available to the muscles and lessens bleeding from small wounds. The person breathes more deeply and the heart beats faster when this system is active. Consequently well-oxygenated blood flows more rapidly round the body. Sympathetic nerves act by releasing two emergency-response hormones, adrenaline and noradrenaline. These closely-related chemical messengers, as well as causing the visible changes as already described, result in invisible chemical changes in the blood which prepare the body for physical activity. This mainly consists of mobilization of the two fuels used by muscles, sugar and fat. Sugar is stored in the liver as animal starch, called glycogen. This is a molecule, shaped like a tree, and is built up by the liver from glucose units in times of sugar surplus after meals. Adrenaline saws up the glycogen trees and pushes the constituent glucose logs out into the blood stream, which carries them to the muscles. There they are either used immediately or converted to muscle glycogen for later use. The rise in blood sugar which adrenaline causes may be an important factor in the relationship between sugar diabetes and atheroma.

Fat is stored as neutral fat which is laid down not only just beneath the skin, but in almost every part of the body. It is called neutral fat because it is made up of a base, glycerol, neutralized by three molecules of fatty acid. Each neutral fat molecule can be visualized as a letter E. The vertical part is the glycerol and the prongs represent the fatty acids. Adrenaline, and more especially noradrenaline, mobilize these fat reserves by splitting the neutral fat into its acidic and basic components, free fatty acids and glycerol, which then pass out of the fat cells into the blood stream. The free fatty acids can then be used as a source of fuel by any of the muscles in the body, including that muscular pump the heart. In fact the heart is the only muscle in the body that can't take a rest throughout its working life of up to one hundred years or more, beating 3,000 million times during a life of average length. It therefore has to burn whatever fuel comes to it in the blood. Fat as a fuel has the disadvantage that it uses up more oxygen than sugar. This is one of the reasons that when the level of free fatty acids in the blood rises too high, the heart tends to beat erratically and with less force. Also for some unknown reason, raised free fatty acid levels also make the tiny blood cells (called platelets, which are responsible for starting the clotting process) stick together more easily. As well as these short-term effects the free fatty acids which are not used up in muscular activity can be converted back to neutral fat by re-combining with glycerol, or be used to make the dreaded cholesterol. If the blood level of these two fats remain raised over a period of years they can be laid down in the walls of the blood vessels and cause atheromatous narrowing, as already described. Thus the stage is set for a heart attack.

In this way a certain pattern of life, called for future reference the aggressive or type A behaviour pattern, increases the amount of stress hormones, adrenaline and noradrenaline, made by the body's sympathetic nervous system. These stress hormones raise the level of free active fat in the blood to prepare the body for physical exertion which, in the modern urban environment, seldom comes. As a result, the now redundant free fatty acids are laid down in the walls of blood vessels as neutral fat and cholesterol. When the coronary arteries have been narrowed by a critical amount, a final stressful episode makes the blood supply to the heart insufficient for its needs, often due to blocking of one of the heart's arteries by the formation of a blood clot on the roughened vessel wall. The heart then either rapidly stops beating for lack of blood supply to its muscular walls, or suffers painful damage in the part supplied by the blocked artery. The basic theme of this book therefore is that the main cause of the plague of heart disease affecting civilized man is imbalance between his mental and physical activity, resulting in an inappropriate chemical response to the sedentary stresses of modern life. Over a period of years the consequent unnecessary mobilization of sugar and fats leads to narrowing of the arteries supplying blood to the heart, and promotes the formation of blood clots, until finally a heart attack occurs.

2. The urban environment

One interesting thing noticed early on about heart attacks was that they are more than three times as common in people living in cities than in country dwellers. It's worth trying to sift out therefore the factors in the urban environment which increase the risk of coronary artery disease. They could be considered separately as affluence, insecurity, inactivity, and overcrowding, though as in most things one problem overlaps another.

Affluence

Coronary artery disease is mainly a disease of affluent societies. It is rare in underdeveloped countries and decreases in time of war when overall levels of affluence decline. Luxury is largely linked with city living as it takes a city to produce large affluent groups. Cities will also often produce large groups of poor people and keep them living in close proximity to the affluent. This is liable to set up stress reactions in both groups. In the absence of a rigid class or caste system the 'have-nots' are envious of the 'haves' and their possessions. Not only are these seen alongside and therefore in sharp contrast to the 'have-nots' belonging, but advertising relentlessly shouts the differences and deficiencies from walls, the pages of newspapers and magazines, and from television. Today's urban spaceman, it is forcibly pointed out, should not be content with 'a jug of wine, a book of verse, and Thou' – what he needs, the story goes, is an ice-cool, super-fizzy, extra-strong, tall glass of sparkling vino-luxe, with added sweetener. This should come straight from the ice box of his mobile, four-wheel drive motorized, mirrored, musical cocktail cabinet. Books are definitely out as even the flimsiest paper-back outlives its commercial usefulness. A portable colour television has much more style. It also rubs into more people around you that you are definitely one up on them, even if you can't quite hear or see it properly out of doors. 'Thou' should be dressed not just to look pretty but in, or preferably ahead of, the latest style, regardless of cost, discomfort or impractibility, even if it does mean wearing a sequinned fur coat over a mink cat-suit on the beach.

Just enough is not enough! Surfeit in every direction should be his goal. If he doesn't get it he is failing in some way, he is letting his family down and it's all his own fault. If he does not even want these things he is regarded as either mentally abnormal or subnormal or both! This unceasing commercial propaganda is likely to induce not only the desired competitive drive and buying urge for which it is designed, but also a sense of impotent rage and frustration when only a few of these artificially created goals are achieved. These are ideal emotions for producing a steady increase in stress hormone levels with the consequent rise in blood fat levels needed to damage the arteries.

Insecurity
Curiously enough it is among the 'have-nots' who manage to make the transition to 'haves' that the toll of heart attacks is greatest. There are several reasons why this may be. Firstly they have to work harder to make the

grade than those born with a silver spoon in their mouths. As the saying goes:

> *The doors of fame are open wide*
> *The halls are always full,*
> *Some go in by the doors marked 'push'*
> *And some by the doors marked 'pull'.*

Pushing is far more stressful than pulling, as readers of the 'Peter Principle' will know, and the former produces correspondingly more stress hormones.

Secondly, they often feel less secure and drink more, smoke more and live a more riotous life to prove to people in general, and themselves in particular, that they are stronger than the next man. These activities, if maintained over a period of years, have a directly adverse effect on the heart.

Thirdly, the self-made man frequently has to sever ties with friends of his youth as he and his family move up the social ladder. This is not only stressful in itself, but sets him adrift in the treacherous waters of social conventions in a new group which may reject him. Added to these feelings of insecurity is a more intense fear that what possessions he has acquired may be stolen or swallowed up in a financial disaster. As the old Tahitian saying has it: 'The man with a big canoe has a big worry'. He knows what it is like to be without his hard-won affluence, and does not want to be that way again. A man brought up on a mountain doesn't get dizzy looking down, while a boy coming up from the sea may well do.

Such considerations may explain why those fortunate enough to start life with the security and poise given by a University degree get significantly less heart attacks than those who get to the same positions in industry from the shop floor. Also Labour Members of Parliament, whether in Government or Opposition, get more heart attacks than Conservative Members. The reason for this unfair Parliamentary division could either be that the former do take their duties more seriously, or else that they feel less secure, so that public speaking and decision-making involve them in greater stress.

Though a rigidly stratified class system as existed in Victorian times often gave rise to gross abuses of both power and wealth, it did form a stable framework from which people could derive some degree of fatalistic security. There was a 'station' in life in which the fates had placed you, and there in all probability you were likely to remain. If you were of noble birth, barring accidents and infighting among relatives, your social position and wealth were secure. Lords and squires had the security that land confers, hence the title of landed gentry. Merchants generally had several generations of experience in trades that had not changed much for hundreds of years, and where the bottom didn't fall out of the market overnight. Craftsmen had arduously acquired skills, could take pride in doing one job from beginning to completion, and were established in their own guild. Servants and their families derived security from their masters' households. The pecking order was relatively fixed and each person knew his position in it and the function he was expected to fulfil. Even the village idiot had his own lowly but safe place in society. Now, however, he has been made redundant by a few highly-paid professional 'idiots' appearing nightly on television as comedians, and is an example of the many minor talents which could be employed in smaller communities but are inadequate in the larger social units.

What has happened in the last hundred years to destroy this sense of security? Firstly, and most importantly, societies have tended to become much larger. Their members lose their sense of identity and individuality among the masses surrounding them, as Desmond Morris describes in his book *The Human Zoo*. Another of his books, *Intimate Behaviour*, describes how simultaneously many people begin to feel emotionally or even physically threatened by the overgrown societies in which they live. They then almost deliberately 'lose touch' with their friends and become more isolated in a crowded city than they ever would have done in a village community. This withdrawal from physical contact and bottling-up of

29

emotion can induce severe mental stress of the type already discussed in relation to heart disease.

Secondly, in larger societies the idea of having a well-defined job to do and an individual role to play that really matters to the people around you is swamped by sheer numbers. The process is intensified by increasing specialization, as doing only a small part of a job rather than seeing it through to the end, lessens motivation by removing the goal.

Physical Inactivity
The particular problems arising from the diet of affluent Western Man is discussed later in this book. However, it should be mentioned here that, with the exception of expectant mothers, most adults in this population could halve their food intake without endangering their health in any way. In fact it would probably be of equal benefit to both their waist-lines and life-lines. This is because in the very societies where foods, particularly sugars and starches, have become more easily and widely available, as well as more attractive and more concentrated due to effective refining processes, the need for food as a source of physical energy has decreased. In the process of civilization much of mankind's mental energy has been devoted to lessening the amount of physical energy used in everyday life. Beginning with the harnessing of animals so that we could use their muscles rather than our own, the process continued with the invention of the wheel. As it came into use in this country round about the time of the building of Stonehenge, it has been suggested that the name was derived from its full title of 'Welsh Hauliers Energy Expenditure Lessener'. Though some doubt this origin of the word, the device greatly decreased the effort involved in moving loads over-land. It was, however, not until steam and then petrol-driven methods of transport became widely available that the level of physical activity in many people's daily lives declined abruptly.

The trend to inactivity was intensified by several other factors. A greater proportion of the population lived in towns or cities, and took up administrative or clerical jobs. This was part of the process of increasing organization and specialization within a civilized society. By removing the need to hunt for food or cultivate crops, it enabled large numbers of people to take up the manufacturing and service occupations on which our present day consumer society is based. The consequent influx of labour-saving devices both at work and in the home leads the inexorable spiral towards a totally push-button age, where the only muscle required will be a flexor on one finger.

To see how far this progressive paralysis is spreading, let us consider a day in the life of *homo execuens*. Awakened from sleep in which his basal metabolism was depressed both by the sedative he took last night and the electric blanket, his physical exertion before breakfast is limited to pressing the 'off' button on the alarm, the 'on' button on the light and raising his electric toothbrush and electric razor to the level of his face. After a brisk bout of wrestling with the press-open box of frosted flakes, the top of the instant coffee jar, and assorted buttons on the pop-up toaster, and the electric stove, he can face the first big physical challenge of the day—getting to work. The button-operated elevator takes him down the two floors from his apartment to his garaged car. A mere six buttons later he has escaped from the underground garage and is engaged in mortal combat with other commuters fighting to reach the city. Being a virile, competitive fellow, he has a gear knob, three pedals, and above all a horn button to help him enjoy this form of psychological warfare to the full. Shaken but triumphant, he hits the button opening the gate of the office garage only three minutes late. Six car buttons, two elevator buttons, and he is installed at his desk.

The working day that follows provides a further six or seven hours of variable emotional activity. The Company pays him to be competitive, driving, time and deadline conscious. In other words, to display all the features of the Type A behaviour pattern as intensely as he can and for as long as he can. In contrast to this high level of mental effort his net physical effort is likely to be limited to operating the buttons of the telephone, the intercom, and the video terminal supplying him with data from the computer. He may be allowed to walk to lunch, though for maximum efficiency he should have sandwiches and coffee brought to him in the office, and use the time having a tense lunch-hour conference. Any meals taken outside the building should only be highly alcoholic affairs to impress business associates that he can't otherwise tolerate, and to temporarily weaken their powers of thinking fractionally more than his own. After a suitably stressful afternoon, preferably with several good rows with any available subordinates, just to make it clear that he is really earning his money, and to relieve the petty frustrations of life such as the button on the automatic coffee machine jamming, he can at last reverse the morning order of button pushing, and fight his way home through the rush-hour traffic. With his television dinner on his lap, the tired executive can relax in an armchair, the push-button remote-control making it unnecessary to rise to change channels. From the briefcase at his side, he can take, when the programmes all finally become too dreadful to watch any longer, some suitably aggravating reports from the office. If even he admits he is too tired to do any more work, he should read a salacious paper-back to remind him of his matrimonial duty to keep up the National Average. He must be forgiven if he fails in this, as after such a day the erogenous zones are more likely to be thought of as just one more set of buttons!

The Nuclear Family

Unreasonable as it may be, modern Western Man is finding his decline in status within the nuclear family a bit of a strain. It has all been rather too sudden for his mind and body to adapt to. The change really set in about sixty years ago, within living memory. There he was, seated comfortably at the top of the family tree, which was roughly where he had been from the start of the human race. His recipe for success was to keep his wife 'bare-foot and pregnant'. This state of almost complete dependency was maintained by careful training in subservience in girlhood and withholding education wherever possible, or at least directing it along safe channels such as music and needlework. A chain of events then occurred to disrupt this pattern of male dominance. Education became more widespread and broader in scope for both boys and girls. The number of careers open to women gradually increased until even the bastions of professions such as medicine and the law fell before their onslaught. The right of women to vote finally removed them from 'man's chattel' status, and their success was capped by the introduction of efficient birth control. Increased industrialization spurred on by two world wars took more women out of their previously mainly domestic role and gave them the chance to show that they could do more jobs as well as, and in some cases better than men.

It is largely as a result of these changes affecting their status within the nuclear family that more men are being forced to follow the active aggressive Type A pattern of behaviour, previously mentioned in relation to coronary heart disease. It is believed, often rightly, that lack of success in the status-affluence race will cause loss of affection and respect both at home and at work. A dominance struggle often builds up in both places, and the more time and energy put into one, the less there is for the other. In the words of the song: 'A tiger by day, he makes business hum, then winds up at night under some woman's thumb'. These influences are most clearly seen when comparing Western with traditional Eastern cultures. In the West equality of the sexes is accepted, and many families are run by matriarchs. Women are educated, often to the same level, in the same co-educational establishments and expect an equal say in family affairs. Some Western women have even been known to dispute their husbands decisions, and wife-beating isn't the popular pastime it used to be. In the East the majority of women are not educated and are brought up in a strict tradition of subservience to male interests. Also the Eastern male is usually more respected if he avoids anything that looks like hard work, which is regarded as being more suitable for the poor, the illiterate, and women. The less industrialized society makes fewer demands in terms of time-keeping and deadline consciousness, and under the reduced pressure, work rate is more regulated by mood and climatic conditions. Finally, failure and poverty are not so much a social and family disgrace, but natural events ordained by fate. It may be pure coincidence that coronary heart disease is relatively uncommon in the men of the overtly patriarchal Eastern societies.

Overcrowding
There is evidence from all over the animal kingdom that overcrowding causes aggression both within and between species. This is part of a basic survival mechanism which under natural conditions limits the number of animals living in any area to one which can obtain their physical and psychological needs from it. When this number is exceeded fighting breaks out and the weaker animals are killed or driven away,

The principle seems to operate in all animal species. Animals, either as groups or individuals, have an innate sense of the extent of the territory that they need for comfortable survival. To show how far down the evolutionary scale this principle extends, Desmond Morris quotes in *The Human Zoo* the example of the male stickleback, who becomes very territorially minded in the breeding season. If pots of waterweed representing the territories of two such males are brought closer and closer together in an aquarium, display threats change to fierce prolonged fighting. Overcrowded rats also become extremely aggressive towards each other. Experiments with other species of animals show how an increase in numbers in a limited space, even when food supplies are adequate, can lead to over-activity, enlarged adrenal glands and heart disease. Several species of birds, including chickens and captive wild woodchucks, die in large numbers from heart disease when there are too many animals in one enclosure. It was found in the Philadelphia Zoo that heart disease increased in antelopes, deer, monkeys and apes when they were exhibited in groups rather than pairs or individually. Further evidence from primates comes from the fact that arterial degeneration is almost unknown in wild monkeys but is found in about twenty per cent of captive ones. Also in Russia it has been shown that monkeys made 'neurotic' by procedures such as intensive handling after capture, severe restriction of movement, or artificial disorganization of sleeping and feeding cycles, often develop high blood pressure or signs of heart disease after only two or three months of such treatment. The effect of the pressures of a cramped urban life on behaviour patterns was clearly shown in a study of urban and rural monkeys in India. The urban monkeys fought much more often and more fiercely than the rural ones, especially when food was at stake. In contrast to the male dominance usual in this species, the country male often gave way to urban females.

Extending these behavioural studies to man, large differences have been found between town and country dwellers, and people who live in large and small cities. The findings in these sober scientific experiments on sociability fitted in with what you would expect from every-day experience. In the larger cities people were more suspicious, more hostile and more aggressive. They were also more time-conscious, to the extent of not even giving away the time of day to the passing stranger. Actively destructive actions were also more common in big cities. A remarkable demonstration of this was obtained by abandoning two similar cars, with the bonnet open, in middle class residential districts in a large and a small American city. In the former destruction began within five minutes and was complete within eight hours. In the latter the only event was when a passer-by lowered the bonnet to stop the engine getting wet when it rained.

In all, the combination of inactivity, insecurity and overcrowding inherent in the modern urban environment make it more than a little surprising that the men subject

35

to not only these but also added ideological pressures do not succumb as rapidly as the monkeys to stress disorders but linger on to middle age. It's a credit to man's adaptability!

3. Driving and the Heart

Previously I have suggested that driving ambition is one of the most important factors in coronary heart disease. It is no coincidence that the word 'driving' is used in relation to the automobile, which translated means 'ego-chariot'. According to psychiatrist Dr Stephen Black, the car symbolizes and brings out our most aggressive emotions. This 'auto-aggression', as I'd like to suggest it be called, is basic to the mystique of motoring and is skilfully promoted by the manufacturers.

As men usually make the final choice in buying a car, the male motif is enshrined in as many parts of the 'bodywork' as possible at the design stage. The body is made as long and 'cigar-shaped' as it can be for the money, and similar forms are echoed wherever possible in the lights, wings-mirrors and other details. An extreme example of these design principles is seen in the E-type Jaguar. A large, powerful, and presumably potent, engine is put in to ensure that the car can rapidly reach speeds well in excess of the modest legal maximum in this country. To 'go like a bomb' is perhaps a rather apt description for a vehicle weighing up to two tons, laden with petrol, travelling at a speed of around one hundred mph. The raucous, throaty, male engine noise can be made more masculine and low pitched if its voice hasn't broken sufficiently, by bolting on a variety of cylindrical voice boxes. Special care and attention is lavished upon the gear lever to give it both the right anatomical appearance and the right feel. Short, stumpy rigidly erect ones have the greatest emotive appeal and are set on special high altars in the majority of sports cars. Long floppy ones, and, horror of horrors, the emasculated automatic drive, are usually reserved for family cars where the owner is assumed to be past it. The gear knob is an important appendage and in the smarter cars is enlarged and suitably ornate.

Auto-aggressive emblems don't end there, however. Headlights are made larger and brighter to dazzle and outshine the other man. Set between them are the teeth of the radiator grill, bared in a permanent menacing snarl. Could those over-riders be enlarged canine teeth? In spite of the risk of impaling pedestrians, the mascot on the bonnet is usually pointed either in design or significance. Arrows are common here, or a more up-to-date design perfected by Mercedes is the circle with or without cross-wires in the centre, suggesting a gun-sight. Some more patriotic post-war English cars even had model Spitfires on the front to carry the illusion a stage further. The blindly heroic Kamikaze method of entering major roads is still undeniably popular and not confined to drivers of Japanese cars. Warning colours and chromium stripes are also useful devices for reinforcing the biological messages of the motor-car. Red used to be a favourite colour for arousing the emotions of young motorists and their passengers, but since Desmond Morris said rude things about it, its symbolism has come to be regarded as too obvious. Bright yellow, preferably with black areas to make the car more nearly resemble a wasp, has largely taken its place. If you want to be more subtle, orange or jungle yellow are suitably daring. Naming the machine is a vital part of channelling man's aggressive impulses into buying and driving a particular car. The choice usually is made from emotive words under the following headings:

Warriors – Avenger, Invader, Interceptor, Hunter.
Weapons – Rapier, Scimitar, Chevron, Spitfire, Javelin.
Wild Animals – Jaguar, Hawk, Stag, Stingray, Mustang.

This fierce, competitive motoring image doesn't end with the buying of a car. To overcome imaginary rivals it has to be super-charged and filled with 'super-performance' petrol to put a tiger, no less, in its tank. It then must be personalized with a variety of bolt-on and stick-on goodies to make it quite clear to all who dare come near that it is your territory and should not be confused with the million others like it on the roads. Outside, extra lights, badges and aerials with pennants create an impressive effect. Inside, much can be done with stickers on all the windows and leopard-skin covers for seats and steering wheel. A nodding dog or a toy tiger in the rear window serves as a light-hearted reminder that your territory is well-guarded. A shrunken head on a chain or a skeleton on a piece of string is another jolly way of getting the message across to your fellow motorist. In case you should think these examples too extreme and unrepresentative, I would ask you to read some of the advertisements and comments in today's journals and study the behaviour of motorists, particularly after a minor accident or parking ticket had dented their ego. A more clear-cut rage reaction you will be unlikely to find during peace-time in modern man. The road traffic accident figures in nearly all Western countries are also an eloquent testimonial to the power of the motor-car as a weapon of destruction, in many cases exceeding the effectiveness, in terms of total deaths per year, of conventional warfare.

Motor Racing
Motor-racing is to the modern Western World what

chariot racing was to the Romans. The skill, thrill, and
spill with the occasional kill elements are the factors
making this the supreme spectator sport of the times.
It is the embodiment of controlled aggressive behaviour
by virile young men, who are not only spurred on by the
rewards of money and adulation which go with victory,
but also by the tremendous boost that some people get
from the active stress hormone, noradrenaline. This
'kick-hormone', as it could be called, has been shown by
elaborate laboratory tests to accelerate the rate of performance of many physical and psychological tasks. Its
ability to turn people on makes it a self-administered drug
of addiction, like the chemically closely similar ampheta-
mine group of drugs such as 'dexadrine'. The answer to
the question 'What do you do for kicks?' then becomes 'I
find something that gives the right size shot of noradrenaline'.

Just as with other drugs of addiction the tendency is for
larger and larger doses of excitement to be needed to
produce the same hormonal kick. It is a relatively common experience in motor-racing circles for some of the
less successful drivers to take progressively greater risks
to make life, and eventually death, more exciting.

In this connection it is interesting to speculate on
the ultimate extreme of speeding up of thought processes which occurs just before a crash. This gives rise to
the often-described illusion of a rapid kaleidoscopic
action replay of past experiences, mingled with the reality
of the accident seen in slow motion. These sensations
were vividly described by one racing driver who lived
to tell the tale of spinning off the track at over one
hundred mph. Apparently the dreamy, waltzing sensation, mixed with the impression of having all the time
in the world to sort out the slightly tricky problem of
overtaking the car in front while travelling backwards,
was interleaved with several memories of events leading
up to the race. Even the series of impacts as the car
ploughed through bales of straw, railings, bushes and
assorted shrubbery, before finally coming to rest in a
field, seemed to happen in slow motion. It was as though

the mind were a cine-camera, running at a faster speed for the few seconds during which the accident was taking place. Experimental studies of the action of noradrenaline on the brain suggest that a sudden surge in the level of this hormone in the blood, or in the central nervous system itself could result in temporary stretching of the apparent time scale. In support of such a theory is the macabre report that noradrenaline levels in blood measured after death greatly exceed those found in the most extreme stress situations during life.

Another action of this 'kick-hormone', which has already been described as playing an important part in the theory that aggressive emotion in the absence of appropriate physical activity is a major cause of coronary heart disease, is triggering the release of fat into the blood. Indeed, it was a chance remark by a friend of mine, Dr Peter Taggart, who is both a heart specialist and international class racing driver, which led to my suggesting the theory in its present form. In November, 1969, he had been recording the heart rates of racing drivers during the stress of major events, and found it rose greatly in the time between arrival at the starting grid and crossing the finishing line, even if the race lasted for two hours. Often the heart was revving as fast as it could go, about 200 beats per minute. This is faster than one would find in a young man exercising to exhaustion. Though such rapid heart rates are mainly due to the hormone adrenaline, measurements also showed that noradrenaline levels were increased to an even greater extent. His crucial observation, however, was that the racing drivers' blood plasma, clear before the race, became milky after it. This was in spite of the fact that owing to pre-race nerves, they seldom had anything to eat previously. This could mean only one thing – that large amounts of the only type of fat that you can see as droplets in the blood plasma, neutral fat, were being made by the drivers themselves, under the aggressive emotional stresses of the race. It was the missing biochemical link between emotion and coronary artery disease, connecting stress hormones, and the free active fat they liberate, with the fatty degeneration of the blood vessels which causes heart attacks. In this way motor racing not only provided the vital clue leading to a clear cut theory, but it gave the ideal test bed for demonstrating the biochemical effect of intense aggressive emotions. However, before dashing off to the track side and bleeding every driver in sight, a great deal of preparatory work was needed to set up the delicate chemical methods used in measuring the very small amounts of the unstable compounds involved in this chain of events.

The biggest of these problems was measuring the stress hormones, adrenaline and noradrenaline. These fragile flowers of feeling disappear from the blood just a few minutes after the emotion producing them has faded. To catch them anywhere near their peak therefore means taking the blood sample the instant the event is over. Even when in the specimen tube, with special preservative added, the amount which can be measured is halved every half an hour. This means that everywhere you go to collect these samples, a lot of bulky additional equipment is needed beside the usual blood-taking 'gear' of syringes, needles, swabs, tourniquet, bottles and pots. This extra equipment includes a portable centrifuge to separate plasma from red cells, vacuum jars containing carbon dioxide snow to instantly freeze the precious plasma samples, and sometimes even a portable electric generator to power the centrifuge. As you can see, it takes quite a bit of organizing to get such a show on the road. Even when you have snap-frozen the plasma sample to preserve that straight-from-the-vein freshness, there is a total of less than a millionth of a .gram of the stress hormones in a litre of blood, and only one hundredth of that amount in the size of blood sample which can safely be taken from active people. To ensure correct measurement of such minute quantities needs the most sensitive and sophisticated chemical analysers. It is only by extreme care over every stage of the analysis that it becomes possible to express emotion in terms of blood chemistry. Although such methods are only in an early and relatively crude state, they appear to be more useful for getting objective evidence on the relationship between stress and heart disease than the battery of subjective psychological tests usually applied.

The fats in the blood are also extremely perishable, and need a special preservative, being kept in iced water in yet another vacuum jar from the moment the sample is separated. Although there is a greater quantity in the blood, they are almost as difficult as the stress hormones to measure because there is a greater variety. Also, there is the problem of sorting out the neutral fat imported from the diet, from the home-made variety produced within the body, which is the type revelant to this theory. Although the former usually disappears from the blood within eight hours, we found it difficult to keep energetic people like the racing drivers off food and drink all day long. Fortunately, in samples taken from those who were unsporting enough to eat, it was possible to filter off the relatively large globules of dietary fat, and analyse the 'skimmed milk' which was left. Having got these mundane details sorted out, the fun could begin. Armed with all the tools of the stress trade, Peter and I set off for the racing circuits. As one of the drivers actually taking part in many of the international motor races which we studied, Peter was able not only to give many of the samples himself, but also to talk his co-driver, Dr Tony Goodwin, and other fellow-drivers into providing the rest. Without these sixteen good-natured heroes, this study of a real-life stress situation could not have been made.

As stress hormones and fat levels vary so rapidly, most of the blood samples were taken with the drivers still sitting in their cars. This meant setting up shop in the pits, a noisy and confusing place for a peace-loving blood chemist. From there we could leap on our victims, either as they perspired gently on the starting-grid, or as they screeched to a halt in the pits immediately after the race. After seizing the blood sample from an arm vein, what was usually a 200-yard dash to the centrifuge began, because for safety reasons there was no electricity supply in the pits. This personal lap-time on foot to the starter's box or first-aid station was usually several seconds slower than that of the drivers round the track, especially towards the end of a day spent racing backwards and forward between pit and centrifuge.

What did all this leaping about on the circuits of Brands Hatch, Nurburgring, Spa and Mugello show? Well, firstly it confirmed Peter's view that the very high heart rates that he had recorded in drivers from the start to the finish of the races was due to the elements of fear and uncertainty causing a dramatic rise in blood adrenaline levels. This hormone drove the heart so fast that usually the reading on the heart rate meter exceeded that on the speedometer.

Secondly it showed that the chain of biochemical events predicted in my theory did at least take place during the extremely aggressive mental stress of motor racing. Noradrenaline levels were doubled immediately before the race and were often more than quadrupled by the end. These hormonal changes were reflected in the skin colour of the drivers, who appeared pale and anxious before the race owing to the small blood vessels in the skin contracting because of the high adrenaline levels. After the race, noradrenaline dominates the scene and the skin blood vessels dilate. This is known to racing drivers as 'getting a glow on'. If the car has broken down, the driver is left red with rage. If it hasn't he is flushed with success. Either way, the hormone levels returned to normal within about twenty minutes. Free fat in the blood was also greatly increased before, and for up to an hour after, racing. This chemically very active type of fat is central to the theory, as not only does it go on to form neutral fat and the dreaded cholesterol, but it could in theory directly cause the deposition of fat in vessel walls. The experiment also showed that even moderate increases in stress hormone levels were sufficient to cause a maximum rise in the amount of free fat present. This was encouraging, for it suggested that we might well find similarly large rises in the less extreme emotional situations, of everyday life.

Another important find in this study was that, as the

amount of free fat in the blood declined, so the amount of neutral fat increased. This suggested that the former was being converted to the latter, so that the results could be expressed on a time basis as a series of mountain peaks. The first, tall, sharply-pointed one represents the hormone levels. This rises rapidly at the start of the event and falls off equally abruptly afterwards. The second mountain, showing alterations in the amount of free fat, rises steadily to reach its peak at the end of the events, and goes back to resting levels about an hour later. In doing so it crosses the up-swing of the neutral fat curve. This increases gradually after the stimulus that gave rise to it, reaching a peak after an hour, but remaining raised for two to three hours or more. Cholesterol levels were not shown to rise appreciably in the racing drivers on the day of their races. However, it is a slow-moving fat which was shown by other studies to rise twelve to twenty-four hours after emotional stress, and to remain at a high level for several days. It is important to understand the sequence of changes and their timing as shown in this study of the blood chemistry of racing drivers, because the hormonal and fat responses have been found to be similar in a wide variety of other active, aggressive stress situations which we have studied. Also, it suggests that a few intensive bouts of such emotion during the day would be likely to maintain continually raised blood fat levels. Lastly, having established this pattern of responses in such an extreme situation, it is possible, using suitable safety precautions, to study the effectiveness of medicines used to prevent these reactions. If they succeed under these conditions, they stand a very good chance of doing so under less trying ones.

From the racing-driver's point of view, it seems unlikely that they damage their hearts by subjecting them to these brief episodes of stress, as the emotional relief obtained by this abreaction process appears to last for several days, and could well counteract the short-term effects described. It is the overall emotional climate that counts rather than the freak storms which are, nonetheless, relevant to the theory.

Driving in Traffic

For the reasons given at the beginning of this chapter driving usually brings out the worst in people, in the form of actively aggressive behaviour. Apart from the risk of immediate death or injury in an accident, Peter Taggart and I were more interested in the short- and long-term effects on the heart of the auto-aggressive emotions aroused by driving in London traffic.

For several years Peter had been pioneering techniques for carrying out continuous monitoring of the heart's electrical activity, known as electro-cardiography or ECG for short. Previously such readings were taken using large and cumbersome equipment, with the patient lying quite still in a hospital bed. Using a newly developed radio-ECG, a whole fresh range of studies on the heart's performance under various emotional and physical stresses became possible. The equipment consisted of two metal discs stuck to the chest wall, with wires attached to carry the minute electrical impulses produced by the beating heart to a small radio-transmitter the size of a cigarette packet. This could be slipped into one of the subject's pockets, and the whole arrangement was both comfortable and unobtrusive. Indeed, after wearing it for some time, like James Bond and his shoulder-holster, the subject used to feel naked without it. The special radio-receiver tuned into the narrow frequency range allowed by the GPO could pick up the signals either from inside the car, or from outside it at ranges up to 300 yards. The former system was used for traffic drivers, and the latter for racing drivers. After amplification the signal showed up on the dial of a heart-rate meter, and could be recorded on one track of a twin-tape recorder. The other track was used for a simultaneous running commentary on events occurring during the drive. In the later experiments we also did blood tests before and after the drive, as with the racing drivers, to measure the changes in the stress hormone and fat levels. Though the subjects were driving their own cars on familiar roads and mostly said they felt relaxed and were not hurrying to get anywhere, there were definite signs of mild to moderate emotional stress during the tests. In healthy subjects this was mainly indicated by an increase in heart rate from the resting level averaging about eighty beats per minute, up to levels between 110 and 150 beats per minute during the drive. Apart from one near-accident, which for a short time produced a heart attack pattern on the ECG of a perfectly fit young woman, the most marked changes were seen during over-taking. It seems as though, when the driver puts his foot hard down on the accelerator, the body responds by injecting more of the stress hormones into the blood. The resulting release of free fat into the blood, as shown by the chemical tests, is equivalent to the action of the throttle, and may lead to oily deposits accumulating in the engine. Unfortunately, except possibly for exercise, a de-coking system for the heart has yet to be discovered.

In subjects who had previously had heart attacks and continued to drive regularly afterwards, the effects of driving on the heart were even more spectacular. Some of these post-coronary drivers' heart rates went as high as 180 beats per minute, racing driver standard. Over half showed abnormal electrical activity on their ECG, the patterns suggesting that their hearts were under considerable strain. Two of the subjects even developed frank heart pain, angina, during the drive, and two more went into heart failure and needed prompt medical treatment. All this happened in people who had had heart attacks and had been warned by their doctors about avoiding undue physical exertion, without the equal or greater dangers of certain particular types of emotional exertion, such as driving, being mentioned.

How to live with your car
If you have a 'heart', don't drive. This may be extreme advice for some coronary cases but it seems to be the moral of the story when you look at the rapid heart rates, kinky ECGs and raised hormone and fat levels in this group of drivers. There are a few who must drive to

live but almost certainly there are many more who drive to their deaths unnecessarily. Many of these hard-driving characters are very successful in their businesses, trades or professions, and could afford to pay a chauffeur or taxi-driver to take them to and from work. Failing this, they could take a little extra time and combine walking and public transport or even cycle on the less lethal roads. Women on the whole make their motoring less competitive than men, and up to late middle age have mysterious biochemical defences against stresses which would turn men's blood quite milky with fat. Until then, it seems only fair therefore to let a woman take the wheel whenever possible. Certainly drivers who have had a heart attack should ensure that the premiums on their life policies are up to date before embarking on a motoring holiday. This is particularly applicable to those going on the Continent where unfamiliarity with the roads combined with the richly moving experience of the vivacious, thrusting motoring style of, for example, the Italians (especially when encountered on a hot summer's day) can push the strongest heart to the limits of its emotional tolerance.

What can the younger, healthy driver do to lessen the effects of the psychological disease of motor-mania on the heart? His best chance seems to be to become prematurely aged, in a motoring sense, as soon as possible. Like man, the motorist passes through seven ages. At first the learner, lurching and stalling in the instructor's car. Then the examinee creeping round the hurdles of the test course. Next the lover, revving like mad and wearing down the back springs with acceleration and other antics. Then a duellist, envious of the larger cars, sudden and quick in overtaking, even at a roundabout. If he survives this he enters the optimal age of the advanced motorist in a comfortable saloon with rounded surfaces inside and out and full of safety devices. On retirement the car usually shrinks as much as the shanks that peddle it. Finally the motorist ends his days without license, without tolls, without parking tickets, without anything. The point of reciting this 'strange eventful history' of the motorist is to stress that the sooner a man reaches maturity in his motoring, the better for his coronary arteries. This includes the avoidance of unnecessary competition on the road and adoption of the view that it is better to travel safely than to arrive in a rage. By coming to look on the car as essentially a motorized arm-chair, one's pattern of motoring behaviour tends to improve. The addition of a radio to play music, which soothes the heart within the savage breast, and the realization that an automatic drive does not significantly lessen the masculinity of its owner, both help to make life on today's crowded roads less of a strain on the driver's heart. The Institute of Advanced Motorists approach to driving has a lot to recommend it in the prevention of both accidental and cardiac deaths.

One of the reasons stated for car manufacturers' support of motor-racing is the claim that it has resulted in improved reliability and safety of cars on the road. On the reliability score this has probably improved little since the 1930's, as many well-made vehicles from that era prove daily on the roads. Present-day planned obsolescence often shows itself as frequent breakdowns from the delivery of a new car onwards, and few remain in good working order after the first three years. The alleged benefits of marathon races such as the Le Mans 24 hour race have had little relevance to everyday motoring.

Of the benefits to safety produced by motor-racing, disc brakes are the most frequently quoted example. These are undoubtedly a big advance in motor-racing design, where over-heating of brakes is a continual problem. Under ordinary road-driving conditions, might not the benefit of discs be outweighed by their leading to over-confidence in braking ability, especially under wet and slippery conditions? I would suggest that any safety advantages which have been gained from motor-racing are more than outweighed by the dangerous illusions it incites that driving is a competitive sport; to use a British oil ad, that you should put 'heart' into your car; and lastly, that road vehicles which can go at over double the legal speed are either necessary or desirable. The true skill in the deadly art of motoring really lies in surviving both its immediate and long-term effects.

4. The Heart at work

As the majority of men spend the most active third of their lives at work, and it is there that life-long behaviour patterns are established, it is less than surprising that some jobs carry a higher coronary risk than others. Whether these jobs choose their victims or the other way about is difficult to decide. The fact remains that even when you balance up the factors of urban living and the sedentary nature of some occupations, those which have in addition the elements of sustained competition, erratic emotional demands, insecurity and irregular hours, often involving a great amount of travel, can combine to make a heart attack the foremost occupational hazard.

In research into the causes of coronary heart disease the job factor is usually relegated to a one-or-two-word definition, such as company director or sales representative, which often serves to obscure, far more than it illuminates, the true inter-action between a person and his employment. It tends to block further thought on whether the individual likes or hates the job, is good or bad at his present level of activity, works hard or takes it easy, and generally whether he is winning or losing the complicated, ritualistic battle for economic, social and, above all, personal survival.

Similarly, when carrying out tests on the heart and on blood chemistry, subjects are usually investigated under what are for them highly abnormal conditions, totally removed from the everyday surroundings in which they 'live, move and have their being'. By attempting to strictly define and standardize the conditions for the performance of these tests in hospital, doctors are in fact applying hospital or laboratory stress tests, to which the patients react with a varying mixture of anxiety and anger. It is the doctors who see the patients 'in the wild', the general practitioners, who come nearest to the root of the problem. The game warden has a great advantage over the zoo keeper in differentiating normal from abnormal patterns of behaviour in wild animals in their natural state. Similar principles apply to the study of what can be considered as basically a disorder arising as a reaction to environmental stress. At the same time, these doctors who glimpse the whole patient and can find so many clues suggesting the origin of the condition, lack both the time and intensely detailed scientific backing needed to prove the case in the medical courts that govern traditional thinking on the subject. In spite of this they recognize only too well the trail of events leading up to a heart attack. This is not because the coronary candidate is a frequent attender of his surgery, one of the always-ailing, 'never-well' twenty per cent of a general practitioner's practice that take up eighty per cent of his time. Quite the reverse. They are usually the 'never-sick' group who seldom visit him, for the simple reason that they are go-getting people, so wound up in their work that they feel they haven't time to be sick. From their employer's point of view they are often model employees, being hard-working and having remarkably little time off sick, particularly for minor illnesses such as colds and 'flu. There could well be a chemical reason for this as, spurred on by large doses of the self-administered drug noradrenaline, the coronary-prone individual drives himself on, priding himself on his toughness.

When he does finally get an attack, the typical coronary victim will apologise for troubling the doctor, but if he could just have something to relieve the 'indigestion' pain, he'd be back to work straight away! If, on the basis of your examination, together with the characteristics of the pain and what you can learn from his family about his pattern of living, you suggest that he may have had a heart attack, he is likely to strongly deny it. To prove his point, if he can still stand, he will probably want to drive to the hospital even if it is twenty miles away for a 'proper' check-up. Call an ambulance and he'll sue!

At the hospital, following his first coronary attack, the patient's reaction to his condition can follow one of three courses. Firstly, especially if the attack is mild, he continues to deny that it was a 'proper' coronary, at worst a slight heart strain, and more likely just a figment of the doctor's imagination. In this case he returns to his former coronary-provoking way of life as soon as possible until he does get a 'proper' one. Like a motorist ignoring a caution for speeding, he rushes on all the faster to a major and perhaps fatal accident.

The second reaction is one of overswing. Brought face to face with the terrible reality of a major illness affecting literally one of the most vital organs of his body, he suffers an emotional shock from which he never recovers. A vicious circle is started, often in hospital, and is sometimes intensified by the doctors and nurses looking after him. After the traditional and very necessary period of bed-rest immediately after the attack, this type of patient views himself as, and eventually becomes, a permanent invalid. He is then obsessed with the avoidance of any exertion, particularly physical. He also clings to a strict diet and as many magic potions as he can get hold of, in the form of anti-coagulants, blood pressure lowerers, water-passers and sedatives to charm his troubles away. Thus his life and range of activity narrows down and he gets progressively weaker until he is of little use to his family, his employer, or even himself.

Thirdly, and hopefully, the patient takes his first coronary as a timely warning and learns enough from the experience to avoid getting another one. After leaving hospital he has a one to two month convalescent period during which he continues the process, begun in hospital by the doctors and social workers, of analysing the pattern of living that led him so close to death. With the insight gained, and a programme for gradually and progressively increasing his physical activity to a high level, he is then ready to return to work. It is here that his employer can greatly aid his recovery by neither overloading him immediately he sticks his head inside the office door, nor, more importantly, by treating him as a permanent cardiac cripple, and worse by invaliding him out of a job. After all the man may have worked his way into a coronary while fighting the company's battles, the heart attack being a sign that he was trying too hard. He probably had a good work record before and is likely to have one again if given some initial encouragement. Indeed if, as a result of the attack, he has learned to channel his competitive drives into those areas of his work where they are really needed, he may be both a more pleasant and more effective associate than before.

The stresses of work as experienced by different people are of course influenced by suitability and adaptability. Just because you have a job which is given a special label doesn't mean you are under the same degree of stress as others nominally in the same situation. Bearing this in mind, I would like, rather than list again the factors which one would expect to be operating in various jobs, to tell you about what is actually found when you look at people at work.

Accountants

This was one of the first occupations in which the links between work-stress and blood chemistry were studied. Fifteen years ago two American doctors, Rosenman and Friedman, unable to make sense of the dietary theory of heart disease, carried out a simple but highly effective piece of research. They interviewed by questionnaire a wide range of executives and a group of doctors treating heart patients. If they had wanted a 'commercial' for the theory that a competitive driving pattern of behaviour was a major cause of heart trouble, they could not have chosen better. Seventy per cent of both groups chose this factor, more than ten times as many as those favouring either anxiety or dietary causes. They then look around for a group of people having marked peaks in the pressure of their work. Accountants appeared to be the ideal group as there is a sharp deadline for them at the end of the tax year. During the four months leading up to this, their working week may more than double, increasing from thirty hours in the summer and autumn to over seventy hours during the 'spring fever' of work.

The findings were dramatic. Monthly blood samples showed consistent and often large rises in blood cholesterol, together with much more rapid blood clotting during the period of intense work. Moreover, the timing and size of these changes closely followed the accountant's subjective impressions of how much strain he was under. Other factors which were measured, such as diet, weight, and amount of exercise, were constant throughout the study. This is important as it provided convincing proof that emotional stress could be directly linked with measurable changes in the blood of a type likely to contribute to getting a heart attack. Indeed, one of these forty middle-aged accountants who had been under very severe work stress during the previous week emphasized this point by suffering a fatal heart attack early in the study.

As mentioned in the chapter on the fall and rise of the emotional stress theory of heart disease, these American investigators then went on to define more sharply the go-getting, competitive, time and dead-line conscious pattern of behaviour strongly associated with heart attacks, and showed the associated differences in body chemistry. Not only did the competitive type A individuals manufacture more stress hormones than the more easy-going type B individuals, but they had higher blood fat levels as well as more rapid blood clotting. This large-scale study of San Francisco business men has provided a vast amount of detailed evidence relating behaviour patterns in Western society to heart disease.

Clerical Workers
In Sweden, research into the physical consequences of the stresses of everyday life is a highly-developed industry. The leading research centre in that country is the Laboratory for Clinical Stress Research in Stockholm, whose head is Dr Lennart Levi. Among the many situations studied by this tireless and prolific research worker during the past ten years, was that of varying the method of payment for a job. On two alternative days, invoice clerks were paid piece-wages over and above their usual salary according to how much they could increase their output above the average rate. This incentive scheme nearly doubled their speed of processing invoices, but did in most girls cause slight feelings of rush and physical discomfort as well as increased fatigue ratings. Marked rises in the output of the two stress hormones were recorded on the two 'piece-work addition' days as compared to two 'salary-only' days. The increase in the 'drive' hormone, noradrenaline, was most pronounced in the afternoon sessions of the 'piece-work' days, whereas the increase in the 'anxiety' hormone, adrenaline, was greatest in the morning sessions of the same days.

These hormonal changes, occurring with even such a brief and self-chosen increase in work load, gives some support for the idea that highly competitive piece-work may cause some people to over-work, and thus undermine their health. If, like the accountants, this group had doubled their hours of work as well as their rate of work and kept this up for several months rather than just two separate days, the associated increase in stress hormones should have been quite spectacular. The likely physical consequences are described in the next study of industrial work.

Additional disadvantages of the piece-work system of payments are the tendency for the quality of the work done to fall off, the temptation to disregard safety regulations for the sake of speed, and hostility arising between workers because some are able to earn more than others. In these ways excessive competition may prove unhealthy both for the individual and the organization in which he works.

Industrial Stress

A second study from Sweden represented industrial stress. This was rather more Machiavellian in design. It involved seizing thirty-three middle-aged, healthy but breakfastless males at seven o'clock in the morning, thrusting a tube into an artery in their arm and then getting them to pretend they were factory workers. The job on which they were supposed to concentrate, after this somewhat trying start to the day, was to sort according to size, 2,000 closely similar ball-bearings. In the two hours allotted for this work, they were subjected to loud machinery noise, flashing lights and to cap it all were given two written messages to say they were slow and careless. Now whether this happy band of workers were reacting to the job or to the investigators we may never know. However, the combination did manage to produce a moderate rise in stress hormone and blood fat levels. Blood pressure and heart rates went up in the subjects under study also. These increases were absent in a control group of volunteers spared the work period, and allowed to listen to soothing music instead.

Any minor criticisms of this study are in no way meant to detract from the extreme importance of such projects in finding optimal conditions for work, but illustrate the difficulties encountered in investigating the complexities of every-day life.

Bus Drivers and Conductors

In this country the classic study on heart disease as an occupational hazard was carried out on bus drivers and conductors working for London Transport. These were rounded up in their hundreds, bled and medically examined twice with an interval of five years between. Soon very interesting differences between the drivers and conductors were noticed. The drivers had both higher blood pressures and cholesterol levels than the conductors, and suffered nearly twice as many heart attacks. The most commonly advanced explanation of these differences was that the physical effort of walking round the bus collecting fares was protecting the conductor's heart. On closer examination, however, it seems this may be an over-simplified view. Most of a conductors' time is spent standing rather than walking and the effort of climbing the stairs is unlikely to raise the pulse of any save the most overweight conductor by more than a few beats per minute. Like other groups who are on their feet for a large part of the day, such as shop assistants, they may develop varicose veins, but the occupation is not generally thought to guarantee a fine physique. Certainly they could not be classed in the moderate or hard manual work category.

What is more probable is that some other aspect of a bus driver's work is putting him in a high-risk situation. This could well be the mental strain and aggravation of driving through traffic all day, responding like one of Pavlov's dogs to the tune of a bell ringing once for stop and two for go. It will be interesting to see what happens when the jobs of driver and conductor are combined in the one-man buses. Certainly early experience in South America where the *'dricons'* of one-man buses have the extra incentive that they are paid according to how rapidly they can complete the route, suggests that the risk of doing the two jobs is additive. In view of the work already carried out, the field is wide open for a follow-up study of this new combination of risk factors, particularly if the latest pocket ECG equipment and biochemical measurements could be used to monitor the men at work.

Taxi drivers are an even more stressed group and might repay study. Not only are they 'loners', but they tend to be more competitive than bus-drivers as their wages are higher, but far less certain, as well as being dependent on individual effort. Many of them can and do work longer and more erratic hours. The way in which frustrations build up during the taxi driver's day is illustrated by a description given of a frequent scene inside one of their tea-cabins. Each 'cabby' is shouting at another and to emphasize what he is saying drums on the side of the cabin with his elbows. After about a quarter of an hour of this tension-releasing 'abreaction', they emerge refreshed, having returned to basal expletive level. Unfortunately, these sessions cannot be entirely effective, as the male coronary ward at the Charing Cross Hospital in the Strand was almost entirely filled most of the time by taxi drivers.

Pilots

Since aeroplanes were first made, flying them has been regarded as a stressful occupation. This was confirmed in terms of increased stress hormone production during investigations carried out soon after the Second World War. The study of stress reactions to flying aircraft is now a major industry for the Civil Aviation Authority and Royal Air Force medical establishments in this country.

Such investigations have shown that there is a high level of emotional arousal, with often more than double the resting stress hormones released throughout the pilot's time at the controls. As would be expected, there are marked peaks of heart rate up to 150 beats per minute on take-off and landing, especially under difficult conditions such as cross-winds or at airports surrounded by hills. Heart rates up to 170 beats per minute were described in Swedish pilots flying F105 fighters, while in link simulators rates over 130 beats per minute were rare. This illustrates a basic problem with such simulators that though they have been developed to the point where it is claimed they can 'make trained pilots cry', extraneous factors present in every-day flights such as operational fatigue, disturbed biological rhythms due to time zone changes, extremes of temperature and humidity and interpersonal conflicts, are not super-added. Also, existing flight simulators are intensively used and rarely available for research purposes. For these reasons it might be preferable to extend in-flight research studies whenever possible. Pocket-sized twenty-four hour ECG recorders are available, which the pilots could apply and operate themselves. Changes in blood fats could also be recorded before and after flights of different durations and at different times of day and night to find the least stressful conditions for operating various routes. The effects of flight stress are seen in the fatigue experienced by all members of the flight crew, but most acutely by the pilots. A recent report by BALPA, the British Airline Pilots' Association, suggested that at least three major crashes were because 'the crew apparently flew a fully serviceable aircraft into the ground'. Why should fatigue among flight crews be increasing when hours of duty are in general decreasing? Mainly it appears to be a question of irregular hours disturbing the body's vital rhythms, most importantly those of sleeping and wakefulness. If, due to changing time zones or working widely varying hours within a few weeks, the hands of the biological clock are put backwards or forwards, it is three to four days before the underlying biochemical mechanisms catch up and are all in step again. Adrenaline, noradrenaline and cortizone from the adrenal gland play a large part in regulating the daily tides of pulse, bloodpressure and temperature, as well as the varying ability of the mind to concentrate and function effectively at different times during the day. These factors have been studied in detail by Dr Lennart Levi at his Institute of Stress Research in Stockholm. There they designed an indoor electronic shooting range on which the effects of fatigue both on the body and its functional efficiency could be measured under prolonged mock-combat conditions. Thirty Swedish officers and corporals whose average age was about thirty and who were attending a platoon-leader training school, 'volunteered' for the experiment. For three days and nights they had to shoot continuously with light beam rifles at small cut-out tank targets which intermittently appeared and moved across the field of vision at varying speeds. Hits and frequency of shots were registered automatically by light sensitive 'photo-diodes' on the targets. For fifteen minutes every three hours there was a cease-fire for a drink of water, two standard sandwiches, subjective fatigue and distress ratings, and a visit to the toilet. Throughout the experiment members of the research staff prevented the subjects from falling asleep or turning away from their task. A wealth of information on biochemical changes resulting from fatigue was gained from this study. As well as the normal fluctuations in stress hormone levels with peaks during the day and troughs at night, these tended to rise during the study particularly in the more tired subjects. At the same time, as 'fatigue' and 'distress' ratings increased, performance both in terms of number of shots and number of hits showed drastic step-wise decreases. Although very similar impressive and detailed evidence has been gained from studies on industrial workers on changing shifts, and it has been found that repeated forced reversal of night/day activity cycles shortens the life of several species, including flies, there is a remarkable reluctance to apply these findings to the life of flyers.

On the basis of these studies two remedies appear at least worthy of trial, preferably on a combined basis. One is for the airlines to regularize the hours of work as far as possible. The other is for aircrew to lower their fatigue levels by improved physical fitness. Regularity of hours of work is probably the more important factor. This could be achieved by shift work or limiting the duration of flights. Shift work is deservedly unpopular because most of the time off, as well as the first days on duty, are spent acclimatizing to the time schedules at home. The alternative is to have a two-shift system, both of eight hours duration, say 08.00 to 16.00 and 16.00 to 24.00. This would avoid the over-night 'grave-yard shift' period of 24.00 to 08.00 when the body's activities are generally at their lowest ebb, and performance is impaired. With effort, people can function with moderate efficiency for short periods even in this phase of their day/night cycle. It means forcing the pace by using the 'afterburn' provided by the stress hormones, which is better kept for true emergencies. The airlines will probably reply to this suggestion that it is uneconomic to use such expensive machinery and facilities for less than two thirds of the day. The same arguments have been applied to computers and even the chemical analysing machines in hospital laboratories. There are times, however, when considerations of both health and safety have to override those of cost-effectiveness.

In addition the lives of those on the ground would be considerably improved by even more complete restrictions on night flying than at present exist. There are at present air-liners which can get you almost anywhere in the world within an eight-hour period. Perhaps one of the greatest attractions of Concorde would be its ability to cover vast distances in a reasonable working day and hence relieve pilot fatigue on the longest hauls. The Trident crash in which thirteen doctors and an equal number of their families and friends were killed on take-off from London Airport in June 1972, has brought home to other members of their profession the inadequacies of the present methods of monitoring and maintaining the health of aircrew in a way few other tragedies could. The disparity between the vast cost of airliners (Trident £4m, wide-bodied aircraft, e.g. Boeing 747, £12m, and Concorde £18m), their maintenance (£250,000 per annum for one of the smaller airliners), and the amount spent on training each pilot (£150,000), when compared to the expenditure on ensuring the fitness of each person on the flight-deck (£50 per annum), has become a matter of general public concern.

The economic facts of death in even a single-seater fighter crash were pointed out in a study of stress reactions in pilots of the Royal Swedish Air Force carried out over five years ago. Loss of a pilot and his high performance aircraft then cost approximately £120,000 and this is likely to have doubled by now. Such figures formed the basis for the not unreasonable statements made in that article that 'There is in modern society no other professional training that can compete with the enormous costs of pilot training. Trained operational aircrew are *per capita* the nation's most valuable man-power.' The vastly increased financial loss and risk to the lives of up to five hundred passengers in one crash, not counting the possible casualties on the ground, puts civil air-line disasters on a yet greater scale of magnitude. Not only are pilots very valuable, they are very vulner-able to coronary heart disease. Examination of the Registrar-General's figures for this disease shows that group 192, which includes aircraft pilots, navigators and flight engineers, has one of the highest heart attack rates. Further, a medical study group of BALPA reported early in 1973 that 111 of the 236 pilots, i.e. nearly half, who retired prematurely on medical grounds between 1964 and 1971, did so because of diseases of the heart and circulation. The report went on to say that this in-creasing trend could be controlled, if not reversed, if pilots ate and smoked less and took more exercise. You may notice these themes crop up once or twice in this book.

Unfortunately, experience has shown that this excel-lent advice for all high-risk coronary groups is unlikely to be acted upon unless it is re-inforced by an intensive health education programme which needs to be detailed in both its explanations and recommendations. There is considerable scope for bringing medical examinations of aircrew out of the age of the horse-drawn carriage, where most of the currently used techniques originated, into the era of space-age technology. This particularly applies to newer methods of checking the heart's action, and measurements of fats and other biochemical parameters of fitness in the blood.

As a method of preventing cardiovascular disease, exercise appears to offer the greatest scope as a positive health measure likely to be attractive to this positive group of people. For over 2,000 years physical exercise has been regarded as the natural antidote to emotional stress. In the dialogues of Plato, Timaeus states: 'Any-one engaged on mathematics or any other strenuous intellectual pursuit should also exercise his body and take part in physical training.' He adds that 'By such moderate motion he can reduce to order and system the qualities and constituents that wander through the body according to their affinities.'

The case for increased participation in physical recreation, even if only as an enjoyable pastime, has been well made more recently by Dr Roger Bannister on behalf of the Sports Council. A feeling of increased well-being, lessened fatigue and improved sleep regularly accompany carefully graded courses of exercise. Decreases in both cholesterol and triglyceride were observed in senior officers in the American Air Force who undertook such training. Lowering of these blood fat fractions has been reported in the majority of regular exercise training schemes where they have been measured, providing dietary intake of sugar and fat were constant.

The provision at major airports of suitable facilities such as a gymnasium and swimming pool might rapidly repay the cost involved by preventing premature retirement of at least some of the thirty pilots disqualified annually on health grounds, as well as being an added social attraction.

If British airlines wished to become pioneers in safeguarding the health of their aircrew, as they have in other aspects of air safety, they could initiate prospective studies of the already-mentioned indices of cardiovascular health. The utility of these in preventing and treating disease would need to be assessed over a three to five year period, in relation to the existing statutory tests. On a 'no-detriment' basis the results of the individual measurements would only be available to the pilot concerned. This feedback of information would enable him to assess his own level of fitness more accurately, and to judge for himself the influence of factors in his life with favourable or unfavourable effects. Such tests are unlikely to produce hypochondriasis in pilots for they, above all people, are aware of the increased safety of monitored systems. Also, as the great English physician Osler observed more than half a century ago, 'It is not the nervous individual who suffers heart disease, but the robust ambitious man, the indicator of whose engines are always set at full ahead.' Though perhaps not originally meant in the aeronautical context, it appears a particularly appropriate description of the type of person likely to take up flying as a career.

As a group of men exposed to an extreme form of modern sedentary stress, perhaps these airborne executives should be the first to be offered the most up-to-date methods in the detection and prevention of this modern epidemic. They have been dealt with at length because they illustrate so well the many ways in which work can affect the heart.

Public Speakers

Accustomed as they may be to public speaking, for many people this is a most stressful event. Several factors decide how anxious the speaker is. Firstly, there is the size of the audience both in terms of numbers and their real or imagined superiority. From personal experience, as far as numbers go, it seems to obey the law of diminishing returns according to a roughly geometric progression. The subjective rating for audience size seems to be 2, 4, 8, 16, 32, 64, 128 and 256. Accordingly, the anticipation of talking to over a hundred people is about four times greater than talking to eight. The points on this scale where you start getting anxious and, at the other end where you stop caring how many more might be present, obviously varies widely according to whether you are an introvert or extrovert, how sure you are of your words and above all on your previous experience. In spite of this, many people, particularly the more creative and imaginative, remain racked with anxiety before every major speech, however many they give. Most learn to cover up, with varying degrees of success, but the alarm bells still jangle inside the body.

What are the speaker's secret fears? These might be described as how to make a fool of yourself in six easy lessons. To start with he might 'dry up'. As those who have experienced it will know, this is a very literal expression and is the reason why most lecture halls and interview rooms provide glasses of water. The sympathetic nervous system is very effective at turning off the flow of saliva in such stress situations. This formed the basis of a simple but supposedly infallible lie detector test used in India for many centuries. At his trial, the accused person was made to take a mouthful of sacred rice off a sacred leaf. The charges were then slowly read out to him, and after a pause for contemplation, he spat the rice back onto the leaf. If the rice was thoroughly moistened with saliva he was presumed innocent, but if it was dry, he was found guilty.

The other form of drying up is where you forget everything you were going to say. This has been known to happen on occasions to even the greatest orators, who found themselves temporarily at a loss for words. The amnesia is common with many types of anxiety situation, and especially in examinations, can cripple both the written and the spoken word. Experimentally, it has been found that novice parachutists, just before they jumped from the aeroplane, couldn't remember nearly as many of a sequence of numbers as they could when standing safely on the ground. This unremarkable finding may be explicable in terms of high levels of adrenaline in the blood, as specific stress-blocking drugs, but not sedatives can lessen or in some cases abolish the effect.

Doctor's you may be surprised to hear, are just as liable to stage fright as any other people. Even though they are taught as students to communicate and discuss their work in both big and small groups, the majority are not the garrulous extroverts that popular films and television programmes make them out to be. As a further exercise in losing friends and acquaintances alike, Dr Peter Taggart and I set out to see what happened when a range of people from medical students to professors, stood up to give a talk. In accordance with our theory that you shouldn't do experiments on other people that you wouldn't do on yourself, we were our own guinea-pigs on many occasions. It became so much a habit that we began to feel improperly dressed if we went to speak without having either a tape- or radio-ECG recorder in our pockets and plasters on our arms from the blood tests.

The results were dramatic. The heart rate of the speakers, whether experienced or inexperienced, rose to anywhere between 120 and 180 beats per minute, averaging out at about 150. This is as fast as many people's hearts go when doing heavy physical work and yet the subjects were standing still. As with the traffic drivers, the ECG tracings showed the kinky waves usually associated with a heart attack. As many of the subjects were hale and healthy students and doctors in their twenties, it is safe to assume they weren't about to drop dead on the spot. This finding on its own was a valuable piece of research as it showed that anxiety alone can play havoc with the appearance of the electrical activity of the heart. Such effects of adrenaline, which we found in increased amounts in the speakers blood, can make interpretation of a very nervous patient's ECG almost impossible. Fortunately the special stress-blocking drugs described later were shown to be able to calm the heart down even in this rather extreme situation, and make both the rate and ECG tracing as normal as it should be in perfectly healthy subjects. These drugs didn't seem to impair our oratory in any way. Rather they had the effect of one or two whiskies, removing some of the nervousness and its unpleasant symptoms such as palpitation and the 'shakes'.

In the group of heart patients that we then went on to study, these drugs had an even more beneficial effect. These people, who ranged from high-powered business executives haranguing their firms' annual conferences, to senior engineers apparently lecturing on how to make concrete aeroplanes, showed some of the most erratic ECG tracings so far seen in any of these studies. This explained the frequent occurrence in speakers of the true heart pain known as angina, and even full-blown heart attacks. Such events are especially common in after-dinner speakers, where the food and wine lure blood away from the heart and brain.

It was in the heart patient that the stress blocking drugs

were most effective. Again they made the rate and rhythm of the heart more normal and at least partly calmed the electrical storm. They also prevented the rise in blood fats seen in both the healthy and heart cases. This normally occurred because of the action of noradrenaline, released to help the person cope with this particularly stressful situation. The amount of this stress hormone increases as the speaker gets more confident and aggressive. This 'turns on' the more extrovert performers, as is demonstrated by the dynamic stars of the stage, who only 'light up' in front of an audience. They then change from their often rather depressive, morose selves and become a mass of all-singing, all-dancing activity. It seems as though they need this noradrenaline 'kick' even more than they need the money. This may explain the multiple 'positively last' appearances of many well-to-do actors and actresses. An additional effect of the consequent rise in blood fats is that the body burns more of them and its heat production goes up. Phrases such as 'warming to your theme' and getting involved in a 'heated argument' could be references to this mechanism.

One difficult situation which arose during this research on public speaking was when one of our post-coronary subjects stood up in a large cold hall in St Albans to give his favourite talk on how, thanks to the miracles of modern heart research, his life had been saved. As he spoke, a faint and erratic, but to the doctors in the audience unmistakable, blipping signal began to come over the loud speaker system as a background to his words. It sounded very much as though his heart was doing its own last tango, and from the expression on his face, his cardiologist sitting in the front row of the audience appeared to think so as well. Somehow the radio-ECG transmitter he was wearing during the talk was broadcasting to the loud-speaker system in use in the hall, instead of just to the receiver and tape recorder set up in a nearby room. Anxious notes and puzzled glances passed up and down the row of people sitting beside him on the platform. Carried away by the exuberance of his own verbosity, he was obviously not to be deterred from finishing his full fifteen minutes' worth of prepared speech. So forcefully was he speaking, we decided he could do without the microphone, and to silence that hectic heart-beat, we switched off the loud-speaker system. He finished his talk in grand style and later said he felt 'great' now he had that 'off his chest', even though it had brought on his angina.

This determination of heart patients to prove their toughness at all costs is both their greatest strength, if channelled to self-help with active treatment, and their greatest weakness if unhealthy outlets for this intense 'drive' continue. The same patient, for example, when we next saw him said he had taken a motoring holiday which he ended by driving down from Scotland over-night. Heart patients who take the attitude 'I'll do this if it kills me' too often and too soon have to pay just that price.

Television Performers
This is an interesting occupation from the point of view of the intensity and duration of the stresses involved. Except possibly for teachers and university lecturers, whose jobs are unlikely to rapidly disappear if they don't get their talks quite right, there can be few groups whose livelihood depends on such brief bouts of public performance. 'You're as good as your last show' is the motto in this industry. Certainly on live shows, news, discussion and topical programmes, this sense of urgency and inability to 'cut and shoot again' dominate the mood in a television studio, both on the floor and in the control room.

It was a fascinating opportunity to find just how great these strains really were when the *Tomorrow's World* team suggested doing a live twenty-minute programme on the theory of heart attack disease outlined in this book. The plan was to take a day-long look at the life of a television reporter from the time he got up in the morning to the live programme as it actually went out in the evening. This piece of *télévision verité* was regarded as a typical piece of BBC narcissism in some quarters. For all that, it did provide interesting experimental results on high performance television personalities in action.

Mike Rodd, at twenty-eight the youngest reporter on the programme, was the one studied in the greatest detail. He was the noblest bleeder of them all, having samples taken before breakfast, on arrival at the studio and before and immediately after the show. This heroism served to show a steady rise in blood fat during the day, reaching a peak immediately after the 'live' show. Similarly, that was the time when the greatest increase in noradrenaline was found. Also, under the action of adrenaline his heart rate showed a rise from an enviably slow rate of sixty beats per minute when he was starting the day, to about one hundred during the walk to the studios. By contrast, this went up to 120 during rehearsal and finally averaged 150 beats per minute during the evening performance before an estimated ten million viewers.

Similar rises in heart rate and blood fats were seen in his fellow reporters, James Burke and William Woollard, though the pulse rate of the doyen of television reporters, Raymond Baxter, never quickened to above 120 beats per minute. Increasing experience and confidence often lessens the heart rate response due to adrenaline released because of anxiety and uncertainty, but the blood fat response due to noradrenaline 'drive' remains unchanged. The speed with which the heart responds to an emergency was shown by the jump in heart rate seen almost exactly ten seconds after the television camera cut to each person.

Not content with allowing us to make pin-cushions of their arms and tune into their hearts, Mike Rodd and James Burke took the well-tried stress-blockers previously given to the public speakers and racing drivers. Apart from feeling a little more relaxed than usual, they noticed no effects. The heart and blood chemistry responses to this intense form of stress, however, were almost entirely abolished. Mike Rodd's heart rate stayed firmly below 110 beats per minute, and was at about ninety for most of the show. James Burke's was similarly lowered during his performance, but broke through when speaking to some glamorous fashion models afterwards. It was a relief to find there are some things even drugs can't suppress.

From these examples of some of the increasing multitude of jobs with a lot of mental stress but little physical activity, we can see how our work can influence our heart and blood chemistry. Sometimes, if one is aware how much anger and frustration can increase blood fats, it might be possible to steer out of rather than into some conflict situations. There are a multitude of much-read but little acted upon books of business relations. Dale Carnegie's *How to Win Friends and Influence People* is an early example, and *How to Win the Business Battle* by Eric Webster a later and more humorous one. Business management courses, which have become so fashionable recently, might include at least one lecture on 'Biochemistry and the Boardroom'.

Firms which demand that their executives should rotate rapidly and continuously round the earth, breaking all known biological rhythms as they go, should not be surprised at the number which go into eternal orbit at an early age. Though it keeps the pension fund healthy, it doesn't do as much for the recipients.

The typical coronary case is a work addict. This addiction can be useful to himself and the organization he serves if kept within the limits set by health and offset by physical antidotes, especially exercise. In excess it can prove as fatal as any other drug. To live for your work may be an admirable ethos. To die for it would seem to be both unnecessary and uneconomic.

5. Home is where the Heart is

There is no doubt that your home life can affect your heart at least as much, if not more, than your work. At home you create an environment which more closely mirrors your overall life-style than your surroundings at work. For example, at home the most common arrangement is to choose one person, and live with her for better or worse for the rest of your life. Perhaps some of those rough patches on the walls of your arteries could be described as 'domestic blisters'. The time you are at work is mainly spent paying for the time you are at home. Also, on average, most people are at home three to four times longer than they are at work, so home influences operate over longer periods. A consistent finding in studies of blood fat levels in individuals over periods of months or years is the influence of events in the home, especially on cholesterol. Accountants, as mentioned in the previous chapter, showed variations in cholesterol level with intensity of work, but doubled these rises during periods of severe domestic upheaval such as divorce.

Another American, Dr Rahe, looked at the pattern of events in people's daily lives in relation to major illnesses, especially heart attacks. He did this by getting a large variety of people to rate a wide range of factors according to the 'intensity of stress' which these caused. This is the scale which 400 Americans gave as corresponding to their experiences in life. It is given in full as it is a very fair summary of the relative importance of many of the stresses of Western life.

Rank	Life event	Mean value
1	Death of spouse	100
2	Divorce	73
3	Marital separation	65
4	Jail term	63
5	Death of close family member	63
6	Personal injury or illness	53
7	Marriage	50
8	Fired at work	47
9	Marital reconciliation	45
10	Retirement	45
11	Change in health of family member	44
12	Pregnancy	40
13	Sex difficulties	39
14	Gain of new family member	39
15	Business readjustment	39
16	Change in financial state	38
17	Death of close friend	37
18	Change to different line of work	36
19	Change in number of arguments with spouse	35
20	Mortgage over $10,000	31
21	Foreclosure of mortgage or loan	30
22	Change in responsibilities at work	29
23	Son or daughter leaving home	29
24	Trouble with in-laws	29
25	Outstanding personal achievement	28
26	Wife begin or stop work	26
27	Begin or end school	26
28	Change in living conditions	25
29	Revision of personal habits	24
30	Trouble with boss	23
31	Change in work hours or conditions	20

Rank	Life event	Mean value
32	Change in residence	20
33	Change in schools	20
34	Change in recreation	19
35	Change in church activities	19
36	Change in social activities	18
37	Mortgage or loan less than $10,000	17
38	Change in sleeping habits	16
39	Change in number of family get-togethers	15
40	Change in eating habits	15
41	Vacation	13
42	Christmas	12
43	Minor violations of the law	11

On this scale you can see that death of the spouse was the most stressful event recorded and rated one hundred units. Divorce rated seventy-three units and loss of employment only forty-seven units. A 'life sum' was then calculated for a large number of heart patients and healthy people. It was found not only to correspond with their urinary stress hormone levels on a week-by-week or month-by-month basis, but also to their liability to coronary thrombosis. Usually the crisis occurred several months before the attack, suggesting a cause-and-effect relationship. On this scale you can see how events at home affect people far more than events at work. In particular, that bereavement is a major cause of coronary deaths, the other partner in a marriage dying soon after their spouse, is not only a commonly held impression, but is supported by a considerable amount of medical evidence. Again these deaths are often due to heart attacks occurring six months to a year later, and have been widely recognized as 'broken heart deaths'.

Children also can expect to carve their marks on their father's arterial tree nowadays. Apart from using an increasing part of the family income to keep them in the style to which they are accustomed, with plenty of new clothes, toys, sweets, comics and varied entertainments, the modern cult of the child demands that they should be

both seen and heard at all times. They are cooped up
with adults for larger parts of the day as living units
and the open spaces surrounding them decrease in size.
Television also plays its part in generating the idea that
the young are the most important people, and in diminishing the regard for parents. Finally, rather than being
apprenticed in his father's trade when he would learn to
respect the parental skills and position in that trade, the
son is more likely to go into a different and sometimes
more highly paid occupation. This produces friction and
hostility within the family, which together with the increasing independence of women, throws additional
strains on the heart of the head of the household.

The part women may play in deciding whether or not a
man will get a heart attack is very hotly debated among
doctors and psycho-analysts. Some cardiologists, like Dr
Peter Nixon in this country, feel that it is possible for
socially or financially over-ambitious women to nag
their husbands' coronary arteries narrow. Others may
do it from a sense of being trapped by children and
domestic routine, regarding these as part of the unfair-
ness of life towards the fair sex. They feel cheated of
opportunities compared with their husbands. This could
be the origin of the saying that 'behind every successful
man is a woman telling him he's wrong'.

The opposite view is expressed by Dr Daniel Schneider,
a New York psychoanalyst, who has written a book
entitled *Psychoanalysis of the Heart Attack.* In this he
suggests that, like governments, men get the wives they
deserve, and that women do not have the power to cause
heart attacks unless the men involved use them in a
certain sick way. Examples of such men, and the types of
women they tend to marry, he gives under the points of
his 'coronary character compass'.

Mr North is described as a quiet, passive yet cultured
man who is not fit by character or stress-resistance for
a rat race in which the human rat really bites. He has
considerable ability and big dreams to go with it. However, he is constantly being cheated and defeated and as
a result becomes quietly enraged. Like his dreams his

sleep is short-lived, and he is something of an insomniac. In his early forties he gradually develops high blood pressure and suffers a coronary attack or stroke as this inward gall erodes arteries all over his body. Physically, he is described as a short, thick-set and hairy mesomorph type. His life situation is beautifully summed up in Peter Ustinov's book *The Loser*. Mrs North is generally quiet, intelligent, long-suffering, devoted to her husband and plays little part in leading him down the northern route to the coronary valley of death.

Mr South by contrast is married to a domineering woman, usually from a brilliant and wealthy family. Though big physically, often over six feet tall and 200 pounds in weight, he is submissive to women, especially his mother. Coming from a well-off background and having a good scholastic record, he succeeds early in his chosen career. In middle age, he characteristically kicks over the traces of his profession and develops ill-founded artistic pretensions in the direction of writing or painting. Lacking talent, they fail miserably, and end up hating their life in general and their demanding ambitious wives in particular. In Dr Schneider's words, this 'Oedipus Enraged' in his paranoid delusions of grandeur 'floats silently down rivers of rage southwards to a lake of tears'.

Mr. East is a short, trim, robust endomorph. A self-made dynamic, go-getting individual, his coronary may have been preceded by a duodenal ulcer some years ago when he was experimenting with how hard he could drive himself. Anxiety and insecurity resulting from his deprived background can result in excess adrenaline release, and either directly by causing spasm of the intestinal blood vessels, or indirectly by other associated nervous and hormonal mechanisms, lead to ulcers. The uncertainty, and fear of ridicule, which plagues this otherwise 'lion-hearted' individual, can lead to further insecurity with his marriage. Although his wife is patient, sympathetic and good-humoured, she is inclined to see the funny side of his predicaments. Unfortunately, this otherwise delightful trait of hers crops up just when, in spite of chewing like hell, he suddenly finds he really has bitten off more than he can chew. As he can't blame her, he alternates between raging at himself and at the incompetence of other people.

Mr. West, a tall thin ectomorph, is often very versatile and genuinely gifted. Though he get his coronary later in life, usually in his early fifties, his rages start earlier in life, usually with almost maniacal temper tantrums in childhood. During these attacks he literally 'sees red' as the noradrenaline storm in the blood makes him go purple with rage. Then even the blood vessels in the eye dilate under its action, and put a red filter in front of the retina, causing a reddening of the field of vision. To compensate, he develops massive self-control during adolescence, and learns to wear a smiling mask to cover the underlying snarl. Having both sadistic and masochistic elements in his make-up, he elaborately builds himself in his married life a trap of sexual anarchy.

As it would be impossible to better Dr Schneider's description of Mrs West, it is best given in full: 'She has a valiant and flashing martyr's complex; it shines out of her on all occasions as if she were a neon woman of push-button, luminous self-sacrifice. In her youth she is apt to be pale, lovely, seemingly tender. This type of woman is forever embittered and never encouraging except when it appears that her husband is about to be publicly acclaimed for some achievement large or small. Then she puts on her tender face, as though taking it out of a jar of cosmetics. To her social group, she appears smiling, tolerant, the very soul of understanding, and the best type of wife for a gifted man. Once the guests have gone, she becomes sharply hostile; the tender face again becomes contorted, critical, even vicious. Their husbands will not uncommonly say: "Her viciousness is a knife in my stomach". In certain circles there is a Madonna-like variation of this type of woman; she goes on a campaign for religion, and sometimes succeeds in breaking her husband down into a religious pulp.' In spite of his Herculean efforts to placate her she is never satisfied. Alberto Moravia described this type of woman as a 'wardrobe', comparing her with Mr West's probable dream woman, the light and frothy 'egg-whisk' type, known as a *frullino* in Italy. Appropriately enough, Mr West is in many ways the model Western coronary-prone male. His life is outwardly perhaps the most successful, but inwardly is the most dominated by anger and frustration. The intensity of his drive and determination to succeed verges at times on the suicidal, his eventual heart attack being the last self-destructive act of an angry man.

The emotion was vividly expressed in a poem of Dr Earl D. Bond, the dean of American psychiatry, quoted by Dana L. Farnsworth in the book *Staying Alive Under the Incentive System*.

WITHOUT LOVE

Love's substitute, ambition grew.
He worked all day and grudged his sleep.
At times he worked the whole night through,
Such toil as made the angels weep.

And when he reached his pinnacle,
The goal to which his labour led,
He faced the inadmissible
And put a bullet through his head.

Why then does he not get his coronary attack earlier in life? The answer probably lies in the fact that his energy overflows into physical restlessness, which keeps his muscles partially active and reduces his weight, both of which have a valuable protective action. Also he is usually too busy and too dynamic to be a glutton, and so keeps down the amount of body fat which can be flung into the bloodstream during his regular rages.

Of the four coronary characters described, Mr West is the one whose wife probably plays the greatest part in bringing on the illness which results from the almost volcanic forces of rage which build up inside him and destroy his blood vessels. He has been well characterized by Dryden as:

A fiery soul, whch working out its way,
Fretted the pigmy-body to decay

Escaping from the frustrations of marriage into the arms of another woman doesn't appear to help much either. Though statistics on this point are understandably hard to come by, the general opinion of doctors is that a relatively large proportion of coronary attacks occur during extra-marital sex, presumably with a true *femme fatale*. Looked at dispassionately, there may be several reasons why an away match may be the last. Firstly there is the time element in the life of a 'two-timing' man. He is constantly trying and failing to be in two places at once, and is likely to end up as the rope in an emotional tug-of-war between two dissatisfied women. One of the penalties of a double life appears to be that you live only about half as long.

Another factor setting the scene for a heart attack might be the intensity of effort and excitement in a man sampling forbidden fruit rather than the home-grown variety. Eager to please the other woman and to prove his virility, in early or even late middle age, he may attempt feats of sexual athleticism that he couldn't even manage in his youth. It doesn't need Kinsey to report that increases in pulse rate and blood pressure occur during intercourse. As with other forms of exercise, the scale of these is related to the speed of the action, and they reach a peak at orgasm. Intense emotion may heighten these normal physical responses, and set up strains which the heart cannot withstand. Within marriage the activity is likely to be less feverish, and probably even more beneficial than other forms of regular, rhythmic exercise in pleasant conditions, because of the emotional relief experienced by both partners.

Even so, heart pain can come on during the most mild love-making in severely affected patients to the point where fear of provoking the intensely unpleasant sensations in the chest or arms may cause impotence. Fortunately, with increasing physical fitness from other forms of exercise, or by the action of drugs such as the stress-blockers described in the next chapter, this symptom can usually be suppressed to the point where a full sex life can again be enjoyed.

Masturbation as a rival activity should not be allowed to get out of hand. Its emotional content is considerably greater than its exercise content. Psychiatrists say that it is basically an aggressive act towards oneself, usually induced by frustration, as the term 'self-abuse' suggests. The noradrenaline release is therefore likely to be relatively large and little of the consequent rise in blood fats used up in the muscular activity involved. As mentioned earlier, prolonged rise in blood fats can lead to narrowing of arteries all over the body, including the ones in the neck supplying blood to the eyes and brain. Perhaps there is some truth, after all, in the old saying that masturbation can make you blind, or mad, or both.

Turning to other pastimes, any absorbing or satisfying hobby from stamp collecting to bee-keeping can relieve the strains set up by modern living. From a detailed study of the leisure activities of civil servants carried out in this country, the one which appeared to be most effective in lessening the chances of getting a heart attack was home decorating. Whether it was the relatively mild physical activity involved, I rather doubt. More probably it was a combination of actually being at home for long periods at a time, rather than constantly away on business or 'working late at the office', and there being a tangible and pleasing end product. Also, preening of the marital nest is a sign of domestic harmony receiving much wifely approval.

More and more people now tend not to have any active leisure-time activities, but only the passive one of watching television. As many of the programmes show scenes of either real or imaginary strife, Dr Taggart and I thought it might be interesting to see how much of the stress on the screen was reflected in the emotions of the viewers. We assumed we knew pretty well all the answers from the previous research done in Sweden by Dr Lennart Levi, but we couldn't have been more wrong.

In the search for a standard and reproducible method of causing different types of emotional response, Dr Levi had done a great deal of work on the reactions of audiences watching various types of film. In one series of experiments he showed his audience four different films on consecutive evenings. On the first evening they watched a bland natural scenery film depicting beautiful pastoral scenes from various parts of Sweden. Next evening they were shown Stanley Kubrick's *Paths of Glory* which was considered to be agitating and anger-provoking. On the third evening the film *Charley's Aunt* directed by Hans Quest was shown and produced suitable merriment. Lastly the by now slightly sated film watchers were revived by Mario Bava's gruesome ghost story *The Mask of Satan.*

Though the vampire physician in the last film was very keen on his blood-sucking activities, Dr Levi wasn't, but confined himself to measuring the stress hormones in urine samples taken before and after the film-watching sessions, and recording the subjects' emotional reactions to the programme. The main findings were that people felt relaxed and their stress hormone output went down with the bland film, but the reverse occurred with the other three. The main rise was in the uncertainty-anxiety hormone, adrenaline.

Unlike so much research which involves stating the obvious and then adding figures to prove it, these findings were interesting because of the unexpected uniformity of response to different stimuli. To confirm this, and provide some factual information for psychologists and gynaecologists alike, Dr Levi next turned to a study of the reactions of men and women to sex films. Working in Sweden, it was not difficult to obtain four suitable films. These were separated by bland, natural scenery films dealing with fauna and flora to relieve the monotony of fornication and defloration.

Exposure to this film caused increased sexual arousal in all but twenty-one per cent of the women and four per cent of the men, whom it left totally cold. More of the men than the women reported being 'fairly' or 'very' aroused, but at the extreme of sexual excitation there were a few women but no men. These subjective impressions were reflected in the urinary stress hormone levels where elevations of both adrenaline, related to excitement, and noradrenaline, related to aggression, were greater in the males.

The conclusions drawn from this experiment were that the result favoured Kinsey's suggestion that females are generally less aroused than males in response to visual, as compared with tactile, sexual stimulation.

From this Swedish work we felt confident that the results on television viewers would be similar, though perhaps on a small scale because of the smaller screen. However, we hoped that we could add something by sampling the hormones while they were still in the blood, measuring the changes in blood fat and recording the minute by minute responses of heart rate to a programme covering a wide range of emotions. Also attempts to subjectively assess the effects, as in the BBC Audience Research Department Report 'Violence on television' (1972) have not provided any clear-cut conclusions. It was therefore decided to examine the objective measures provided by biochemical and electro-cardiological changes resulting from such exposure.

Television watching
Ten pairs of healthy men and women watched a pre-recorded television programme, two couples at a time. The subjects fasted for six hours after a light lunch, and separately, in a side room, had a fine tube put in an arm vein for withdrawing the blood samples. ECG electrodes were attached, and linked to a central switching box outside the viewing room by extended leads. The ECG of each subject in turn could be recorded by rotating the selection switch.

The hour-long test programme was supplied by the Further Education Department of the BBC and the study formed part of a programme being made by that department on the social and biological effects of stress. The telerecording was replayed on to a conventional domestic receiver situated in the comfortable, congenial setting of the television viewing room of Moorfields Hospital, High Holborn, from an Ampex 7003 telerecorder unit in an adjacent control room. The subjects' reactions to the programme could be observed through a glass panel between these two rooms. The viewing-room was illuminated by subdued overhead lighting.

The four sections of the programme lasted approximately fifteen minutes each and represented:

(1) *Relaxation:* This control period consisted of a soporific commentary on underwater life, including various types of sea-weed and small marine animals.

(2) *Humour:* To cover a range of comedy, two seven-minute extracts were combined in this section. The first was from a Morecambe and Wise television programme which won a Golden Rose of Montreux Award. It consisted mainly of dialogues between the two comedians. The second featured Eric Sykes in a situation comedy describing an attack on the BBC Television Centre by Red Indians. The aggressive element of humour was evident in the castration threats in the former and ritual mayhem in the latter.

(3) *Violence:* Verbal assault followed by physical assault on a bus conductor by a gang of teenagers. The 'beating-up' was brief and not explicit by present-day standards.

(4) *Suspense:* A very tense situation from the last of a series of Doomwatch programmes, in which one of the heroes is defusing an activated hydrogen bomb washed up on to the end of a pier. After an agonizing and eventful countdown, the last charge explodes and kills him.

Although it might have been preferable to vary the running order, because of difficulty in altering the video-tape, the sections were always shown in the sequence given, with five minute intervals between to allow for the collection of blood samples. This was carried out with as little disturbance as possible and the arm re-enclosed in a paper towel to minimize the impairment of concentration on the programme inherent in this experimental situation.

It was difficult to distinguish any consistent bio-chemical response to the different sections of the television programme. The only change in stress hormones was a rise in adrenaline occurring after the humorous section. Overall, the free fat level rose, and neutral fat and cholesterol fell during the programme. Glucose levels rose after the violence section, and remained elevated during the suspense and second control period.

The most marked change in the electro-cardiographic recordings was a moderate slowing of the heart starting during the humorous section of the programme, and continuing during the violence and suspense sequences. In view of the presence of increased sympathetic activity suggested by the increases in plasma adrenaline, free fat and glucose, more detailed analysis of the ECG tracings was carried out for evidence of increased activity of the opposing part of the autonomic nervous system, the parasympathetic vagus nerve. One such index is the slowing of the heart rate which occurs during expiration.

Analysed on this basis, the ECG recordings showed significant decrease in minimum heart rate and increase in maximum heart rate, resulting in almost trebling of the gap between the two during the humour, violence and suspense sections of the television programme.

Film viewing

The experience gained in the previous study, combined with the previously described work of Lennart Levi on subjects viewing a variety of films, suggested that this medium might provide a more intense stimulus than television. This would be expected from the more all-embracing size of the image presented, the relative unfamiliarity of the surroundings, and the effect of being part of a larger audience. It is not unusual for the managers of cinemas showing films explicitly depicting violence to be required to provide assistance to people suffering vaso-vagal fainting attacks. In extreme cases vomiting and incontinence of urine and/or faeces may occur as additional signs of profound parasympathetic over-activity.

Perhaps to even a greater extent than television, the cinema is under increasing criticism for relying on violence to attract audiences. In view of the cardiac responses to the violent and suspense episodes in the television programme, a modified study was designed to investigate reactions to films of violence currently being shown.

There was a total of 46 visits by 34 subjects to the film *Clockwork Orange* directed by Stanley Kubrick, and twelve subjects went to see the film *Soldier Blue* directed by Ralph Nelson. A dose of one of the β-blocking drugs described in chapter six was given to half the subjects six hours and one hour before they viewed the film in an attempt to separate parasympathetic from sympathetic effects. Having fasted for six hours after a light, fat-free lunch, had ECG electrodes with extended leads attached, been bled and given urine samples, the group of ten or twelve subjects were taken to the cinema by taxi. The group sat in two equal rows of pre-booked seats. An ECG operator sat in the middle of each row and during the pre-film commercials, connected the leads from each person, including his own, into a six position switching box. The leads, lying across the subjects' laps, being covered by jumpers or jackets, were inconspicuous and caused no embarrassment or inconvenience.

By operating the six-position switch on the selector box, which was connected to the pocket-sized ECG recorder, tracings could be obtained from each subject at any desired point in the film. Using a 'Pocket Memo' type of recorder, the sound track of the film could be used to provide a synchronous commentary.

Stress hormone estimations on the urine showed that the adrenaline secretion rate was almost doubled during the film. The rise in urinary noradrenaline level was less marked, however.

Free fat levels were almost doubled after the film in both the unblocked groups with much smaller increases in the blocked groups. Neutral fat decreased in all groups, but the cholesterol and sugar levels remained unchanged.

The ECG recordings, when analysed in the same way as those taken during the television study, showed slowing to well below control values in all groups, especially during the most violent sequences. Except for a moderate degree of slowing in the unblocked females, maximum heart rates remained unchanged. The increase in the gap between the two which occurred during the film in all groups, was more marked in the blocked subjects.

To elucidate the factors underlying the biochemical changes, further hormonal estimations were made in the six unblocked and six blocked subjects attending the film *Soldier Blue*. Increases in a hormone called growth hormone were found, to which the break-down of neutral fat to free fat could be attributed.

The theme of *Clockwork Orange* is that the normal reaction to witnessing scenes of violence is a sensation of sickness, amounting to an aversion. It is suggested in the film that in some individuals a sense of excitation predominates over this aversion, so that they either seek out or create scenes of violence to feed this appetite for excitement.

The main character in this film, Alexander Delarche, is led, in his search for stimulation from violence, to the 'inadvertent killing of a person'. As a test case in the curtailment of prison sentences for violent criminals, he undergoes aversion therapy. This consists of forcing him to watch films depicting extremes of violence and, at the same time, administering anorexant drugs to re-establish the assocation between violence and an intense sensation of sickness.

This treatment is so successful that he is released with a hypersensitivity to violence which makes him helpless in a violent society. The film ends with his abrupt de-sensitization by the mental and physical trauma of a suicide attempt.

A correlation is apparent between the theme of this film and the cardiological and biochemical findings in the people watching the violence it depicts. The vagotonicity of violence even in the relatively hardened medical audience examined in this study is shown by the slowing of the heart and is supported by the changes in the levels of the hormones such as growth hormone.

Other investigators have found that repeated exposure

to films depicting mutilating accidents or operations could lessen the subsequent subjective and physiological responses to similar stress. Most workers emphasize that the effectiveness of such treatments to reduce stress lies not in the initial exposure to the stressor, but in repeated exposure or in psychological terms 'cognitive rehearsal'.

A great deal of research already carried out has consistently shown that violent behaviour can be learned from both films and television as well as real life situations such as Northern Ireland. Like most teaching it is especially effective at an early age, when related to real-life situations, carried out by people with whom the subject can identify, made interesting and exciting, and above all when it is rewarded and encouraged by peer groups. The stimulating influence of crowds and martial music, 'that divine dynamite' in rousing the aggressive emotions and counteracting vagal inhibitions, was well known to military leaders before the American physiologist Cannon described it in 1929. Kubrick reinforces this message by using the music of Beethoven and Rossini to make the violence of the *Clockwork Orange* acceptable. Thus, to increase the audience for violence, the vehicle for it is supercharged with the excitement generated by sexual themes and powerful music, and given a hard gloss of professionalism, enabling the most sordid events to be presented in a brilliant, glittering 'ultraviolent' light.

This study suggested that these objective methods, especially with the addition of β-blockade, could be used to measure the rate of desensitization produced by the portrayal of violence on television and films.

It is perhaps optimistic to expect that this vagally mediated aversion to violence can be allowed to decrease in the population without socially harmful effects becoming apparent. Being 'sick to the heart' with violence may be one of the most effective and necessary forces in restraining man's innate tendency to aggression.

6. Drink, drugs and diet

There is a certain amount of truth in the saying that the way to a man's heart is through his stomach. Western society has a consuming passion – consuming. This doesn't just apply to the consumer durables such as cars, television sets and the hundred-and-one gleaming domestic gadgets with which we litter our lives like jackdaws filling their nest with junk and jewellery.

> *Eastern potentates, so we are told,*
> *Often used to be weighed in gold,*
> *Western man is worth his weight*
> *In baser metal – chromium plate.*

To fit the consumer creed, from birth we are taught, enticed, and encouraged to constantly stuff as much into our mouths as we can. This included not only more food and drink than we actually need, but also medicines and cigarettes. Deep in the brain lies a satiety centre, which once upon a time used to regulate our appetites according to the needs of our bodies. Affluent societies have learned to over-ride this control system for reasons of convenience, commercial profitability and as a means of pacifying minds unsettled by the stresses of modern life.

In his book *How to live with your heart*, Dr Barry Carruthers accurately describes this means of pacification as 'eating to fill an empty heart'. Even though heart disease has taken over from tuberculosis as 'captain of the men of death', I suggest that the main cause is a more modern form of 'galloping consumption'. Examples of the liquids, solids and gases with which we over-fill our bodies and the pills with which we try to compensate for these excesses, are given in alphabetical order.

Alcohol
This has been man's pleasure and comfort from earliest times, through ages when heart disease was practically unknown. Obviously heavy drinking, as well as being fattening, causes the type of troubles at home and at work likely to lead to heart disease, as shown by the large amount of neutral fat in the blood of alcoholics. Except for these extremes, it remains one of the best ways of unwinding the coiled spring of a day's activities, and even getting to sleep at night if you feel overloaded. For most people it is better than any known tranquillizer or sedative and more enjoyable to take.

For those with coronary artery disease, while the excesses limit applies with greater force, it can be a useful aid to treatment. Firstly it can make for relaxation and general lowering of stress hormone levels. This reduces the levels of some fats in the blood, and makes blood clots less likely to form. It also dilates blood vessels all over the body, including those of the heart, and so tends to relieve rather than bring on heart pain (angina).

Anticoagulants
These were introduced with a fanfare of pharmaceutical trumpets in the 1950's as being the answer to heart disease. The advantages were theoretically obvious. Heart attacks, it was said, are due to coronary thrombosis, the clotting of blood within the coronary arteries. Make the blood less coaguable, and your problems were solved.

Unfortunately, it turned out not to be quite so simple. Firstly some people died before you could give them the anticoagulants. Of those that died a large proportion showed no blood-clot blocking their coronary arteries. Also the treatment had to be controlled by frequent blood tests and even then was not free of the danger of causing bleeding anywhere in the body, even in the brain. Finally, while giving heart patients anticoagulants when they were still in hospital did slightly decrease the deaths from blood clots forming in leg veins, it had little effect in preventing further heart attacks once they left hospital. For these reasons, anticoagulants such as Warfarin, which was originally developed as a rat poison, have come to be considered as unsuitable for long term use in treating victims of the human rat-race. In fact they are even losing the battle in that field, as Warfarin-resistant super-rats are making a come-back.

Ascorbic acid (Vitamin C)

Linus Pauling, the Nobel Prize-winner in chemistry, has recently put forward several biochemical reasons why this vitamin might provide some protection against ailments ranging from cancer to the common cold. While this is a rather extreme view, there is some evidence that Vitamin C is linked in some way with the complicated story of heart disease. There are two main points in favour of this idea. Firstly, Vitamin C levels in people with advanced disease of the coronary arteries tend to be lower than those in a healthy group. This lowering is mild, certainly not enough to show up as scurvy, and requires sensitive chemical tests to detect it.

Secondly, it has been suggested on the basis of experiments carried out in Czechoslovakia, that low Vitamin C levels can be related to high cholesterol levels in both the blood and the other tissues of the body. This is because, in guinea pigs at least, Vitamin C deficiency slows the rate of conversion of cholesterol to bile acids, a route by which it is normally removed from the body. Guinea pigs had to be used for these experiments because like humans, but unlike rats and rabbits, their bodies cannot make this vitamin, but have to rely on a supply in the diet. Fresh fruit and vegetables are the main source of Vitamin C in the diet. They are filling yet not fattening and contain a large amount of roughage which again, according to some of the latest theories of Dr Dennis Burkitt, is a sovereign remedy against heart disease and colon cancer alike. Though these conditions are not unknown in vegetarians, it is claimed that they are much less frequent. The emphasis on the freshness of the fruit and vegetables is because Vitamin C is unstable, its breakdown being hastened by heat and light. Lastly, any oils which may be present in vegetables are of the unsaturated variety, which again are supposed to have a cholesterol-lowering action.

For all these reasons, whichever theory of heart disease prevention you care to back, you can hedge your bets by having a diet with plenty of fruit and vegetables in it. Again, according to Dr Linus Pauling, an apple a day is not quite enough to keep the doctor away. Each apple contains about 5 mg of Vitamin C so you would need to eat at least a bushel (200–300 apples) a day to get up to the one or two grams a day level which he thinks likely to give most benefit. Also it becomes rather expensive to continuously take the various pure forms of Vitamin C which are at present on the market, and more work is needed to prove its medical benefits before it can be recommended as a routine preventive measure. For example, Vitamin C deficiency may just be a sign rather than a cause of heart disease. It is, however, a very safe compound to take, and there is no fear of overdosage as being a water-soluble vitamin any excess rapidly overflows into the urine.

Aspirin

This remedy for aches, pains, cold and 'flu is just making a spectacular come-back in the field of heart disease. It has been found to have previously unsuspected biochemical properties among which is the ability to prevent blood platelets sticking together. When platelets stick to each other and to the vessel wall, they release clotting factors and can cause the formation of a blood clot. Just half an aspirin tablet reduces the patelets sticking tendencies for between one and five days. Also deaths from heart disease are considerably lower in groups of people taking regular doses of aspirin, such as those with arthritis. This is not proof positive of its effectiveness, however, as the arthritic sufferers may differ in many respects, especially psychologically, from those without the condition and hence not taking aspirin. However, the suggestion made last year by Dr Lee Wood of the Hope Medical Center, California, that men over the age of twenty and women over forty, should take one aspirin tablet daily, seems worth a trial in high risk groups. The only exceptions are those with aspirin allergy, uncontrolled high blood pressure, ulcers or bleeding disorders, where aspirin would be unsafe. As he says the treatment may turn out to be ineffective, but the cost and dangers are minute, and possible benefits enormous.

Beta-blockers

What on earth would you want your beta's blocked for, you may well ask. To give them their full title, 'beta' refers to the adrenergic beta-receptor sites of the autonomic nervous system. If this doesn't immediately make the action of these compounds crystal clear, try thinking of them as stress-blockers. They act by preventing the stress hormones adrenaline and noradrenaline from acting, rather than preventing their release in the first place. They were first produced in Britain by ICI in the early 1960's as drugs to be used for the relief of heart pain. They proved very effective in many cases, and so several new compounds were introduced, propranolol (Inderal) and practolol (Eraldin), by ICI, and oxprenolol (Trasicor) by CIBA. These three compounds have led the field over the past five years and are basically similar in their action; the last two, however, are not yet marketed in America.

Gradually more exciting effects of beta-blockers are being found than just their angina-relieving ability. As their action was studied in more detail, it became clear that they could slow down the heart and prevent it beating irregularly not only during physical effort, but also during emotional stress. This was seen in the studies on lecturers, television performers and racing drivers carried out with Dr Peter Taggart and Dr Walter Somerville at the Middlesex Hospital, as described earlier. These investigations also showed that other important effects of stress, such as the rises in blood sugar caused by adrenaline and of blood fats caused by noradrenaline could be prevented by beta-blockers. Furthermore, they could prevent blood platelets sticking together and in larger doses lowered blood pressure and even relieved anxiety symptoms. They seemed to approach the ideal medicine demanded of the physician by Macbeth which could:

> *Raze out the written troubles of the brain,*
> *And with some sweet oblivious antidote,*
> *Cleanse the stuffed bosom of that perilous stuff,*
> *Which weighs upon the heart.*
>
> (MACBETH, V, iii, 40)

The 'written troubles of the brain' obviously referred to anxiety and 'that perilous stuff which weighs upon the heart' could only be fat and clumped platelets causing the heavy, pressing sensation of angina.

With these encouraging thoughts, several short and long-term studies of beta-blockers in the treatment of heart disease have started. Before we all dash off to the chemist for our own supplies, however, a few cautionary remarks should be made. Firstly, as with the oral contraceptive pills, no one is yet quite sure what long-term effects on the body drugs with such a wide range of actions might have, even though in the short-term they mainly look beneficial. Secondly, the complete absence of any effect on the full range of mental skills and physical co-ordination in high-performance occupations such as flying a plane, or even driving a car, has yet to be proved.

Certainly the results in tests carried out so far have been largely satisfactory. The small number of racing drivers we tested on an empty track went round just as fast with beta-blockade using oxprenolol, as without it.

Using the same drug, the speakers spoke as well as usual and even felt better than they usually did on such occasions, because of the relief of anxiety. Ski-jumpers studied in Switzerland appeared to jump as well with the drug. However, on psycho-motor tests in the laboratory one group of workers showed a slight decrease in performance and another no change. In a few people who already suffer from asthma, they can bring on attacks. They are also moderately expensive.

In time these β-blocking compounds may reach the stage where they come to be regarded as 'the Pill' for men and will go through the same shifts in the climate of medical opinion as did 'the Pill' for women. After the honeymoon period, when they are regarded as the universal panacea, some infrequent serious side-effects will be found and some doctors may echo the later opinion of Macbeth: 'Throw physic to the dogs, I'll none of it'. The pendulum will then swing back to the more neutral position, that these are very useful drugs when used in the right people with the right safety precautions.

Cigarettes

Smoking certainly causes as many deaths from heart disease as it does from lung cancer, probably more. Heavy cigarette smokers, over twenty-per-day-men, are three times as likely to die of heart disease in general as non-smokers. This can be either from heart failure or coronary thrombosis.

How do cigarettes cause the heart to fail? Nicotine and tars from the burning tobacco leaf distill over in the smoke, causing the fine hairs lining the windpipe and bronchi to become paralyzed for the duration of the smoke. If they are constantly insulted and damaged in this fashion they give up and go away, only to reappear miraculously if you give up smoking for a month or two. If not, it is this type of change in the lining membranes which is thought to go on to cancer. The job of the fine hairs in this membrane is to form a type of 'travelator'. Beating in unison, they constantly waft irritant particles, mucus and any bacteria or dust which may have been inhaled up into the back of the throat, where it is swallowed or coughed out. With this elegant and effective mechanism put out of action by the nicotine, a load of irritant and infected rubbish accumulates in the lungs during the day. Overnight the lungs get a chance to drain downwards and the hairs make a slight recovery, so that in the morning the enthusiastic smoker hawks and heaves and strains to get rid of the phlegm he finds at the back of his throat, modestly and yet almost proudly referring to it as his 'smoker's cough'.

This unbeatable combination of repeated inflammations of his lungs and windpipe, together with increased sputum production from the irritant action of the smoke, and tearing of the small air-sacs in the lungs by coughing, causes two of the most crippling of chest diseases in England, chronic bronchitis and emphysema. These in turn, because of the scarring and destruction of lung tissue, put a heavier and heavier strain on the heart, eventually causing it to fail.

Turning from this harrowing story of heart failure, there are two alternative routes by which smoking may lead to coronary thrombosis. One which has received a lot of publicity in the last year is a theory concerning the gas carbon monoxide which is present in cigarette smoke. This, it is suggested, is absorbed into the blood stream and reduces the oxygen-carrying power of the blood, which in turn could damage the lining of the blood vessels. I personally find this a bald and unconvincing narrative. Policemen on point duty, constantly exposed to exhaust fumes, do not have a high heart attack rate, and neither do gas fitters with similar occupational exposure.

The other, more attractive, theory forms part of the chain of biochemical events leading up to a heart attack along the lines suggested in the first chapter. Some factor in the cigarette smoke, probably the nicotine, stimulates the nervous system and causes the hormone noradrenaline to be released into the blood. This hormone pushes up the blood pressure and mobilizes fatty acids from the body's fat stores. As usual, these acids make the platelets stickier, increase the amount of oxygen needed by the heart and increase the amount of cholesterol and other fats in the blood. Interestingly, the rise in cholesterol during smoking is greater in women than men. All these effects have been proved by repeated experiments over the past ten years, and seem the perfect recipe for a heart attack.

Why, then, when it is clearly recognized and repeatedly stated that smoking causes lung cancer and greatly increases the risk of heart disease, are 40 percent of the men and 30 percent of the women in the United States smokers, and cigarette sales at a record high? Total cigarette sales in the United States are around $5.5 billion, one-fourth the amount allocated for health in the federal budget.

Higher cigarette sales also mean higher revenues from state and federal taxes. The federal government has shown some signs of conscience, however, perhaps partly prompted by the many millions of dollars cost and working days lost from heart and lung diseases caused by smoking. Since the Surgeon General's report on the dangers of smoking on January 11, 1964, money has been budgeted for research and education. In 1972, the U.S. government spent about $2 million on education and $8 million on research. While this in encouraging, it is still less than one-twenty-fifth of the amount spent on advertising cigarettes in the United States.

Cigarette manufacturers are also conducting their own larger-scale campaign to counteract the impression that their products might damage health. By association with beautiful sylvan scenes and outdoor activities such as sailing and athletics, they contrive to convince the population that there is something daring, virile and almost positively health-giving about a habit which is in fact undermining the health of millions of Western people.

This is a pure advertising confidence trick. No sailor worth his salt would light up a cigarette while sailing his racing dinghy. Very few serious athletes would dream of smoking, as they know perfectly well it would put them right out of the running. Why on earth should it be suggested you would want to climb to the top of a mountain in the fresh spring air only to fill your lungs with a form of portable pollution?

There are several reasons why people smoke, and cigarette advertisers naturally make the best use they can of each of them. The main types of smoking have been classified as:

1. *Psycho-social smoking:* This is the way most smoking starts in adolescence, and occurs only in company. It is an attempt to prove maturity, social status and, for those who like king-sized cigarettes and cigars, masculinity. If the smoke is not inhaled, little nicotine is absorbed and the habit remains mild, intermittent and relatively easy to drop. Inhalation allows nicotine absorption and leads on to the other forms of smoking. Health education in schools and universities probably stands the best chance of being effective in this situation.

2. *Tranquillization:* This has been described by Desmond Morris in his book *The Human Zoo* as being a displacement activity, occupying the hands to relieve anxiety and tension. Like the dummy in the baby's mouth, or thumb-sucking in children, it gives what the psychologists call 'oral gratification'. An effective antidote to this form of smoking might be gentle ridicule, such as posters of a man with a baby's dummy in his mouth and a caption saying 'Smokers are suckers'.

3. *Indulgent:* This is smoking taken as a self-administered reward in association with other pleasures such as reading, watching television and eating or drinking. When not engaged in these activities, there may be a gap of several hours without any wish to smoke. The most effective way of helping these smokers to give up is to point out the association, and then separate smoking from other activities. When they feel the need to smoke, going into a cold, unpleasant room and sitting on a hard chair facing a blank wall, should prevent smoking being regarded as a luxury. Another way is to satiate the

smoker by getting him to deliberately double his cigarette consumption for two days and then treble it for two
days. He should then be more than ready to give up completely, just for the relief.

4. *Stimulation:* It has already been described how smoking can cause the release of noradrenaline. This can
actually cause a temporary improvement in performance
or creativity and a re-awakening of interest in a boring
task. In some ways it is the most dangerous type of
smoking because it is used to suppress stress symptoms
and over-ride the warning signs of fatigue. It is at its
worst in stressful situations such as long-distance driving,
and when trying to meet deadlines during business crises.
The combination greatly increases the amount of blood
fat and sets the scene for a heart attack.

5. *Addiction:* This is reached through one of the other
types of smoking, and is almost as pathetic and certainly
far more common than any other type of addiction. The
addict feels physically sick unless he has a cigarette at
least every twenty to thirty minutes from first thing in
the morning to last thing at night. The withdrawal
symptoms he otherwise experiences are because of the
biochemical need to maintain either high brain nicotine
levels or high blood noradrenaline levels. This type of
smoking is the most important to stop and also the
hardest. In spite of attempts to lessen the craving for
nicotine by substituting tablets containing similar chemi-
cals such as lobeline, it often takes an abrupt shock
such as a heart attack to break the addiction. Even then
there is a very high relapse rate.

Three out of four people who smoke try to give it
up, but only one of them succeeds. What can be done to
improve the odds? The wish to succeed can be reinforced
in several ways. Emphasizing the dangers has probably
been pushed to the point where some people will continue smoking out of bravado, using the 'cancer-stick'
to play cigarette roulette with death. However, equating
the booklet of gifts which can be obtained with the

coupons in each packet with the risks of various types of illness which could also be earned, might help illustrate the point. Doctors have set a good example in giving up smoking over the last few years. The results so far are impressive. It has been estimated that the number of doctors whose lives are saved each year equals the output of an average medical school. Most hospitals are now mounting campaigns to actively discourage staff, students and even visitors from smoking. A lot more could be done by doctors, especially general practitioners in strongly advising and encouraging smokers to give up, especially at the times when the illnesses caused by smoking have just been experienced. Many smokers stop spontaneously during brief illnesses and then all the doctor needs to do is to exhort them not to restart.

Finally, it should be emphasized that the only effective way to stop smoking is to cease abruptly and completely. Posting your cigarettes and lighter to your worst enemy might do the trick. Cutting down gradually is sure to cause relapses. Your friends and relatives can help by not offering you cigarettes and by not mocking your heroic and immensely worthwhile efforts.

The old bogey of putting on weight, perhaps due to the lower levels of the fat mobilizing noradrenaline hormone, can be tackled some time after the cigarette problem has been beaten. The risks of being slightly overweight for a few months are far less than the hazards of continuing to smoke. Changing to another brand with lower nicotine and tar levels, according to a league chart issued by the Department of Health and Social Security, is likely to lull people into a false sense of security by perpetuating the myth of a 'safe cigarette'. Most of the brands with a low tar content also have a low nicotine content. As the heaviest smokers are in the 'stimulation' and 'addiction' groups who depend on nicotine and the consequent noradrenaline secretion, they are unlikely to find the low nicotine cigarettes satisfying. Also, there is the danger of people who might otherwise not start smoking, or who might give it up, smoking the 'safer' brands, and then as their need for nicotine increased and the habit gained a stronger grip they would change up to the 'stronger' grades, like other addicts making the transition from 'pot' to 'hash'.

As an example of the techniques which are, I think, unethically used to promote cigarette sales, on the reverse side of the page of *The Times* which gave the tables of nicotine and tar content, was a five-times larger full-page advertisement recommending the league leader. This used every trick in the book. It had two photographs. One showed the open packet beside an elegant coffee cup (indulgence). The coffee in the cup was being layered with cream poured over what was obviously a silver spoon (psycho-social). The companion photograph showed the full range of cigarettes the firm made, including one with more than three times the nicotine and tar content of their best brand. The slogan in two-inch high letters at the top of the advertisement modestly proclaimed the safety of 'the mild cigarette' and encouraged smokers, new and old, to try smoking it. The usual patter about this brand being a 'smooth, balanced smoke', indeed a 'smooth, mild but satisfying smoke' (tranquillization) were followed by the interesting information that 'cool, fresh air is drawn in with the smoke'. With all these features designed to promote our delight and health alike, the final 'added benefit' of gift coupons seems almost too much to ask. The health warning tucked out of the way on the side of the packet is devalued by implication to being just them, the Government, trying to spoil everybody's fun, and as such is almost totally without effect. If the Government were seriously intent on cutting down the health hazards of smoking, it would abolish all forms of cigarette advertising, as it does with other potentially addictive drugs, and prohibit smoking on public transport and in public buildings. Otherwise any money they put into anti-smoking campaigns is largely wasted.

Clofibrate (Atromid–S)

This is a drug which has gained some popularity in the prevention of second heart attacks and treating heart pain. It reduces levels of all the three main sorts of fat in the blood, fatty acids, neutral fat and cholesterol. The results obtained with it could best be described as encouraging, but far from conclusive. The main benefits were obtained in smokers and in reducing sudden deaths from heart attacks. This fits in best with its ability to decrease fatty acid levels, as its benefits did not appear to be related to the reductions in neutral fat or cholesterol. Clofibrate is moderately expensive and the results of trials so far nowhere near sufficiently dramatic to warrant putting apparently healthy people on it as a routine preventive measure. The position was well summed up by a recent conference of heart and circulation doctors and chemists. After several lectures extolling the virtues of Clofibrate, the chairman of the meeting asked those among the hundred experts present who actually took this medicine themselves to put up their hands. Only three did!

Coffee and other beverages

As well as the 'it's what you eat that does it' school of thought on heart disease, there is an 'It's what you drink' school which points an accusing finger at coffee in particular. It gives as evidence such studies as the 'Boston Collaborative Drug Surveillance Program', otherwise known as 'The Boston Coffee Party'. This found that people admitted to hospital with a heart attack drank more coffee on average than those admitted with other conditions, a relationship which did not hold for tea. The results could be taken to suggest either that coffee drinking causes heart attacks, or, alternatively, that it is associated with them in some non-contributory way.

As a cause, there is evidence from Sweden that coffee can increase noradrenaline levels, being another way in which the stimulant action of this self-administered drug can be produced. However, some of the constituents of coffee can interfere with the chemical tests for noradrenaline, so this action has yet to be proved.

On the question of whether it is an indirect association

between coffee drinking and heart disease, several factors have to be considered. Firstly, there is the possibility that the sugar in the coffee might be the link, as suggested by Professor Yudkin in this country. This may play a part, but the difference between coffee and tea drinkers can't be explained on this basis. Secondly, the milk substitutes often used in coffee in America may play a part. The most commonly used are based on coconut oil, which though a vegetable oil, is one of the few which are saturated and so might be expected to raise cholesterol levels. Cigarette consumption too is closely related to coffee drinking habits, as mentioned in the section on indulgent smoking.

Last but not least is the possibility that coffee consumption is higher in people trying to drive themselves on through the types of emotional stress and fatigue which usually precedes a heart attack. English studies show a relationship between tea consumption and heart attacks, but not coffee. Perhaps this Anglo-American division could result from stress driving an Englishman to drink tea and an American to drink coffee.

To demonstrate the principle that you can't win when considering all the things which might be related to heart attacks, even the purest water, of the type low in calcium and magnesium, has received its share of blame. It was found that heart attacks were slightly more frequent in soft water areas than hard water areas. However, it is a bit difficult to imagine, with food coming from all over the country, and the milk or tea or coffee swamping any mineral deficiencies in the water supply, that this is a major factor.

Diet

This is deliberately left till last and dealt with in the length I feel it deserves. Others disagree, so if interested, read their books on the subject.

Probably the main factor in the diet of Western man which contributes to heart disease is its general excess. This particularly applies to sugar and starch, less so to fats, and least to protein. Sugars and starches are the substances which are most easily produced in highly concentrated and palatable forms. Consequently a vast amount of commercial effort has gone into promoting their consumption in amounts which far exceed most people's needs in relation to their energy expenditure. To test the truth of this statement, look at the minute amount of sugar and starch in any effective reducing diet, as this represents the amount of food you actually need to stay alive at your optimal weight.

Manufacturers have found it difficult to cram our lives with a gross excess of dietary fat because on its own, a large amount of fat is nauseating. They have had some success by combining fat with sugar and starches, as in creams, whips and fillings. There are some true cases of fat intolerance and a few rare familial blood fat disorders needing a low fat diet. However, for the reasons given in the first chapter, I firmly believe that excess dietary fat plays little part in causing the majority of cases of heart disease. At a recent meeting of blood fat experts in London, the day was largely taken up with discussing the benefits of low fat diets. In the evening, at the official conference dinner, the menu was:

Pâté Maison
Poached Salmon with Sauce Hollandaise
   (made with the finest butter)
Entrecôte Chasseur with French Fried Potatoes
Soufflé Surprise
Coffee (with cream)

It was apparently thoroughly enjoyed by all the experts present and so it would seem unwise to disagree with their implied verdict on the practical importance of diet.

This overfed Western way of existence has rightly been called 'The Sweet Life'. Rather than give elaborate diet charts telling you in minute and boring detail what to eat and what not to eat, I suggest a simple rule – usually, avoid sweet things. This includes sugar, cakes, biscuits and 'sweets' of both the pudding and confectionery kind. 'Usually' means don't make a fetish of it, as some 'sweets' are far too good to miss. Most of them are just a consumer habit started in childhood. Parents can play a large part in safe-guarding their children's teeth and arteries alike by this slight but important change in the family's diet.

7. The Fitness factor

Up to now I have dealt mainly with factors which in excess can do you harm. Saying 'don't do such and such' is a rather negative approach and overall it will never be a hit. What I would rather leave uppermost in your minds is the thought that getting and keeping fit is a positive measure which can act as an antidote to a large number of otherwise harmful habits. Believe it or not, exercise need not hurt to do you good and can even be enjoyable. If you are a work addict, for your heart's sake try becoming an exercise addict also.

'Our research has revealed' is a favourite phrase with scientists. Using all the latest scientific machines described earlier in this book, including analysers that can measure infinitesimal amounts of hormones in the blood, and gadgets that can transmit the hearts electrical activity from a racing car going at 200 miles an hour to a trackside recorder, we managed to re-discover the ancient truth that mental activity needs to be balanced by physical activity. 2,000 years ago the Greeks recognised this basic human need for exercise with greater clarity than most world authorities do today. They believed that good health could be maintained by a balanced pattern of living. This was the original meaning of hygiene, before it became a dirty word. The essential reasons behind this belief are beautifully expressed by Timaeus in the dialogues of Plato: 'For health and sickness, virtue and vice, the proportion or disproportion between soul and body is far the most important factor; yet we pay no attention to it and fail to notice that when a strong and powerful mind has too weak and feeble a bodily vehicle, or when the combination is reversed, the whole creature is without beauty, because it lacks the most important kind of proportion . . . When the mind is too big for the body its energy shakes the whole frame and fills it with inner disorders; the effort of study and research breaks it down, the stresses and controversies involved in teaching and argument, public or private, rack it with fever, and bring on rheums which deceive most so-called physicans into wrong diagnosis . . . There is one safeguard against both dangers, which is to avoid exercising either body or mind without the other, and take part in physical training; while the man who devotes his attention to physical fitness should correspondingly take mental exercise and have cultured and intellectual interests . . . All kind of diseases therefore should, as far as leisure permits, be controlled by a proper regime of life, and stubborn complaints should not be irritated by drugs.'

Dryden expressed the same idea equally clearly a mere 300 years ago when he said:

> *Better to hunt in fields for health unbought*
> *Than fee the doctor for nauseous draught,*
> *The wise, for cure, on exercise depend;*
> *God never made his work for man to mend*

For the past hundred years the place of exercise in the prevention and treatment of disease has been eclipsed by the wonders of scientific medicine with its drugs, diets and operations. Those who suffered heart attacks were traditionally advised not to exert themselves physically and to 'take it easy' long after the two month period that it takes the heart to heal was over. This advice was based on the fact that exercise can make the heart beat faster. Also, if incorrectly chosen, it can raise the blood pressure, as will be described later in this chapter, and bring on angina or a further heart attack. It was even said that each person had a predestined limited number of heart-beats to last a life time and these shouldn't be squandered on exercise.

However, the 'anti-exertional mavericks' (as one leading American cardiologist once called them) overlooked some other equally important facts. The first is that the heart is a muscle and even after a heart attack can be re-trained and gather strength. If on the contrary it is never again even cautiously 'stretched' it steadily gets weaker. The end result is often a cardiac cripple too worried to stir from his wheel-chair or bed.

Also ignored is the effect of emotion, which as described earlier can make the heart beat just as fast as quite severe physical exertion. The strains of such every-day activities as opening the bowels, especially when made additionally costive by inactivity, can send up blood pressure to greater heights than most forms of exercise which are likely to be recommended to the cardiac patient. In other words, the heart is likely to have to stand up to considerable strain even in a physically inactive life, and so usually needs to be re-trained rather than rested. Slowly we are emerging from the dark ages as regards exercise. Many benefits can now actually be quantified in terms of magic numbers and so achieve medical respectability. Most of the known risk factors in heart disease such as high blood fat levels, high blood pressure, sugar intolerance and rapid blood clotting have been found to decrease in suitably physical training schemes. The subjects also look and feel better, cope more easily at home and at work and sleep more soundly at night.

Best of all, there is some recent evidence provided by Professor Morris at the appropriately named School of Hygiene in London, that civil servants who take even a modest amount of vigorous exercise during the week, more than halve their chances of getting a heart attack. This, added to the often-shown protective effect of physically strenuous jobs, gives sufficient encouragement to recommend carefully chosen and graded exercise for those who wish to lessen their chances of suffering a heart attack. Therefore I shall look at various forms of exercise, some well studied and others not, and try to pick out some of the good and bad points of each. We'll start with the one that first interested me in exercise as an antidote to stress. Previously at school, any form of sport had been a disaster. Cricket balls and footballs slipped straight between my hands or feet and I somehow wasn't built for running or jumping. This, and hours of having to stand around, usually in the cold or damp, acting as audience for those who were good at competitive games, led to early innoculation against sport. My house master's remarks about early nights and plenty of hard exercise being good for a boy was generally considered a rude joke. I emerged from school with two further stock jokes about exercise. One was the saying by Mark Twain that the only exercise he ever took was walking to the funeral of his friends who took exercise. The other was about when you got the feeling you might take up exercise, you should lie down till the feeling wears off. The reason for my conversion to being an exercise enthusiast will become apparent as we go along.

Gymnasium exercises

Over the past three years the Medical Research Council and the Sports Council have together been sponsoring a study of the effects of carefully controlled gymnasium exercise on business executives in the City of London. The City Gymnasium, where these studies were carried out, is run by Alistair Murray, who, as well as being an Olympic weight-lifting coach, is a fully-qualified remedial gymnast. He has managed to combine his detailed knowledge of both the theory and practice of exercise with the ability to motivate people so that they enjoy and therefore continue with their programme of activity. Use of the exercise schedules he had designed several years before enabled the principles involved in improving the strength, agility and all-round fitness of athletes to be applied to unfit sedentary adults. At the same time the study showed that the careful build-up in work-load, avoidance of 'static' exercises, and constant checking of pulse rates, were necessary safety features in the design of any form of vigorous activity for those high coronary risk group. Just how great this risk is, was seen when some of the 'healthy' people wishing to start exercising at the gym were first put through a battery of heart and blood tests. Nearly a third of this group were found to have signs or symptoms of early heart disease and two of them showed signs of actually having had a recent heart attack. However, the care taken to avoid over-exertion was such that none of the 2,000 'healthy' individuals and only one of the 500 'coronary' subjects exercising in the gymnasium over the past five years have had heart attacks while they were active members. The one who did only visited the gymnasium occasionally and died at home some days after he last exercised. As well as showing the safety of this form of exercise, the low coronary attack rate gives an indication of its probable effectiveness in the prevention of heart disease.

Just how are the benefits maximized and dangers minimized? When you enter the gymnasium, the first impression is one of comfort and luxury rather than the spartan simplicity you might expect from previous experiences at school or in the army. It is a warm, well-lit, softly-carpeted room, gleaming with chromium apparatus and with golden frescoes of manly vigour on the wall. Even the music designed to 'soothe a savage breast' is relaxing yet invigorating. New members are asked about any medical condition from which they may have suffered and about their previous level of physical activity. On the first few visits to the gymnasium they do very light exercise, scarcely more than left and right finger raising. They are then taught how to count their pulse at the wrist, checking it with one of the pulse-rate meters around the gym. The exercises proper then begin with fifteen-minute sessions two or preferably three times each week. The aim is to raise the pulse rate to an individually pre-determined zone about twenty beats wide for most of the exercise period, and keep it there with only brief rests between exercises. For healthy people the top of the target zone, above which it is unsafe to let the pulse-rate rise, is usually 200 less the age, e.g. 160 for a forty-year old fit adult, the zone being 140 to 160. Anyone who has had a heart attack starts the exercise game with a 'penalty' of thirty years added to his age. Thus a forty-year-old who had a coronary two or three months ago, starts off exercising in the 110 to 130 zone. Gradually, depending on how both he and the instructor feel he is progressing, he can often shed these penalty years as he reconditions his heart. The design of gymnasium exercise schedules has been very carefully thought out to minimize the strain on the body in general and the heart in particular. Though at first sight the gymnasium has a large number of impressive-looking bar-bells carrying weights of varying sizes, you never see anyone straining as they lift one. This is for the simple reason that the exercises have been designed to involve vigorous repeated movements and not a few maximal ones, and so each person only exercises with weights he can handle comfortably at his particular stage of training.

It is important to know the difference between these two types of exercise. The first is where the load on which the muscles are acting is moved. Then the tension or tone in them stays about the same, giving isotonic exercise (*iso*=same, *tonic*=tone). The second is where the load is not moved. Then the tension in the muscle increases because it does not shorten or lengthen, this being isometric exercise (*iso*=same, *metric*=length). This sort of exercise is generally thought to be positively dangerous to those at risk from heart trouble because it abruptly pushes up the blood pressure and the amount of work the heart has to do. It also stops you breathing, sometimes permanently.

One famous example of this is Sir Winston Churchill who suffered his first heart attack while straining to raise a jammed sash window. Similarly, heart attacks commonly occur in men trying to push their own or other people's cars, particularly in the cold and after a meal. Exasperation, causing noradrenaline and hence blood fat rises, may well also play a part in such situations. Press-ups are an example of an exertion which is mainly isometric, as the body and legs are held in a static position whilst the arms bend and stretch. When the word 'exercise' is mentioned many people automatically think of press-ups. There are two main reasons why this is so. Firstly the exercise is sufficiently unpleasant and undignified to stick in most people's memories for the rest of their lives. If a games master at school, or PT instructor in the army wants to almost literally 'take a rise' out of those at his command, he just has to make them do press-ups. The starting position, flat on your face, puts you at a huge psychological disadvantage to begin with. If you are overweight or weak, you seize up after a few efforts. Even the very fit can be painfully reduced to panting, exhausted wrecks within a minute by this cunning combination of mental and physical torture.

Secondly, it is wrongly assumed that you can judge how fit a person is by the number of press-ups he can do. This is a fallacy, as it is a very limited test of your power-weight ratio; the power in your arms versus the weight of your body. It can be shown scientifically by using the bathroom scales, that when you triumphantly stand poised on your arms you are supporting almost two thirds of your body weight. More alarming still, the thrust needed to hoist yourself into this totally unnatural posture is anything up to your total body weight. If anyone suggested that raising your similarly-sized wife up to arms length whilst lying on your back as many times as you could before you collapsed was a good way of starting an exercise programme, people might justifiably say they were mad. Yet press-ups are included in almost every 'keep-fit' schedule, from the *Sunday Times* Commando Exercises onwards. There are special dangers in press-ups for heart patients. Such near-maximal effort raises the blood pressure considerably, and slows the return of blood to the heart by shutting off the veins, as well as sending up the pressure inside the chest. Also, the chest is fixed in a cramped position by the arms and the lungs can't expand freely. Finally, exercises should be sufficiently pleasant to make the person want to continue. Only the most enthusiastic masochist is likely to go on doing press-ups for many years. In all, this is the perfect example of the very worst type of exercise for unfit adults. As you may by now have guessed, my motto is 'down with press-ups'.

Meanwhile, back at the City Gymnasium, where they are well aware of the vital differences between isometric and isotonic exercise, and press-ups are taboo, the study of Alistair Murray's training system continues. Each session starts with a few light limbering-up exercises, including arm swinging, leg-raising, trunk bending and cycling. The exercise schedule proper then begins and is geared to each person's individual level of fitness at that time. The ten or twelve exercises which are performed for about a minute each, remain the same. However, as fitness increases the weights used are stepped up week by week to keep the pulse rate within the target zone for most of the exercise period, and more repetitions of each movement can be carried out in the time. Starting with a very light bar-bell alone, weights are gradually added until with peak fitness reached after several months steady progression, a healthy 40-year-old will be using weights of up to 30 lbs. This is not really all that much considering many people are two stone overweight and carry round that extra load all day. Each movement is repeated ten to twenty times or more without discomfort and without raising the pulse above the upper limit of the target zone. This could be called the 'daily dozen dozen' or 3-D system. Increasing both the weight and number of repetitions has several advantages. Firstly it enables the work load to be calculated in engineering terms. This enables the individual to regulate his own progress and to see the effect of mental fatigue and leaving off training in reducing his capacity for physical work. It is also useful in charting progress for research purposes, the only accurate alternative being a bicycle ergometer. This machine, where you pedal against an adjustable friction load is boring to train on alone, and mainly gives you beautifully muscled legs. By contrast, the varied routine of the gymnasium keeps up your interest and exercises every part of the body. Also it means you can cram enough exercise into just fifteen minutes two or three times each week, to reach and maintain most of the sought-after advantages of exercise.

The subjective benefits reported by those following this system include looking and feeling years younger, coping better and being more even-tempered at home and at work, and improved sleep with less fatigue during the day. The objective benefits measured within two to three months of beginning the exercises include improved fitness as shown by being able to do three to six times as much work for a given pulse rate, increased mobility of the spine and large joint, and large reductions in all three of the blood fats measured, including the dreaded cholesterol. Some people also showed decreases in blood-pressure. Though on a constant diet except for those considerably overweight, average weight reductions in those following this exercise regime were small. There were some indications though that the amount of body fat was going down and the amount of muscle going up. If this is so it should be very beneficial, as during stress the quantity of fat released into the blood is related to the size of the body stores beneath the skin and elsewhere. If these are reduced and the amount of muscle available to burn them up is increased, there should be less fat left floating round in the blood stream to promote blood-clotting and furring up of the arteries.

Encouraging though these measurable objective bene-fits are to those trying to prevent heart disease and promote physical well-being in the population, they should not be thought to outweigh the subjective ones. Indeed, the psychotherapy of getting away from the office into pleasant relaxing but invigorating surround-ings with pleasant company with which to discuss your successes and problems. It is a form of group therapy, and a constant undercurrent of positive health education is promoted. Even if it does not lengthen life, and there is every indication that in terms of improvement of the quality of life, this and other types of exercise would still be more than justified.

Unfortunately it is necessary to end on a note of caution. There are very few physical training instructors or remedial gymnasts equipped with the detailed knowledge needed to safely design and supervise a programme of exercise for the really unfit adult. Many are tempted to apply programmes suitable for the very young or the very fit to this group, or start unsuitable exercises at too high a work load. Like most powerful medicines, exercise has to be taken with care. It is hoped that national training schemes will be started for training the trainers in this field.

Swimming

Swimming is another form of exercise which when taken non-competitively and under the right conditions is well suited for the prevention of heart trouble. Again it can be made a pleasant, varied and sociable activity in which the whole family can join. It is also a vigorous, essentially isotonic exercise, whose intensity can be varied according to the distance swum and the time taken to do it. Again all the muscles in the body take their share of the work, especially those of the chest and shoulders, and this is a point very much in its favour.

One factor which causes concern when swimming is mentioned as a form of exercise for the unfit is breathing. In the breast stroke this is not a problem because you naturally breathe on every stroke. With the front crawl however, many people only breathe every two or three strokes and this can throw some additional strain on the heart. However, this is a minor problem and it is only when the breath is held while swimming long distances under water that the blood pressure really builds up and the heart slows right down. This is reflex action, similar to the slowing of the dolphin's heart when they dive. In some relatively young swimmers it has, however, proved fatal, perhaps because in the young such reflexes are stronger. However, in the unfit middle-aged person the strain of swimming long distances under water without breathing apparatus is probably best avoided. The temperature of the water is also important in swimming. This was shown by experiments Dr Peter Taggart and I carried out on the cold dip enthusiasts who swim all the year round in the Hampstead and Highgate ponds. Round about Christmas time when the water temperature was somewhat chilly, 7°C, we took blood samples and measured the blood pressure before and after a five minute swim.

Throughout the swim the volunteer's ECG was being recorded by means of a radio-electrocardiograph tucked in the back of his shorts. The transmitter was enclosed in a polythene bag into which the leads connecting it to the chest had been carefully sealed in an attempt to make it water-proof. Unfortunately, on a couple of occasions the sealing system broke down and we were left at the end of the swim with a rather expensive electric gold-fish inside a bag full of murky pond-water. As these machines cost about £200 each we were lucky that it dried out all right. Anyway, we found that when you leap into cold water, or, for that matter whenever you get cold, your body turns on its oil-fired central heating. This is the noradrenaline-triggered blood fat releasing system, in this case used appropriately to provide the extra heat needed by the body. This increase in heat production is very necessary as heat loss in water is fifteen times greater than in still air at the same temperature. Even so, there is a limit to the length of time you can keep your body temperature up. After about fifteen minutes in really cold water your body temperature drops and when it does so, you can swim no longer. Cramp also comes on more rapidly in cold water, especially after a large meal. This may be due to the extra oxygen needed by muscles using fatty fuel.

One of the people who helped us greatly in this research on cold-water swimming was the internationally famous long-distance swimmer Kevin Murphy. He has accomplished many notable feats, including on one occasion swimming the English Channel both ways non-stop. His gluttony for punishment is such that in 1975 he plans a non-stop three-way channel swim, and in 1974 a two-way non-stop crossing of the Irish sea. He swam the latter one way in 1970, although the effort cost the previous two men to try it their lives. In 1971 he swam round the Isle of Wight, a distance of sixty-six miles. 1972 was a quiet year, only rating a swim across a shark-infested bay in South Africa inside what everyone hoped was a shark-proof cage. His big ambition is to swim 100 miles across the North Sea. Like most long-distance swimmers, Kevin is stocky in build and has a considerable amount of body fat for a very fit person. This is both his long-distance tanks, full of fuel oil for energy and warmth and a moderately effective insulator. Though long-distance swimmers anoint themselves liberally with wool fat and olive oil, or Vaseline, before a swim, this provides relatively little insulation. It is mainly for lubrication, to prevent chafing of the skin by clothing as well as helping to repel the jelly fish. Water temperature is about 16° during most cross Channel swims and the ability to keep going is largely dependent on keeping body temperature up. Exhaustion sets in when the body temperature has fallen from 37°C to the critical level of 34°C.

One of the animals best adapted to cold-water swimming is the whale. Being cylindrical, it has the least surface area for heat loss. It is insulated against the cold by its vast layers of blubber, which also acts as stores of high energy fuel. Finally, it has large adrenal glands with the highest concentration of noradrenaline known in any animal. This enables it to switch its heat production on and off at will according to the temperature of the water in which it happens to find itself.

Where do these fascinating bits of incidental information fit in with you and I taking a cold plunge? Firstly, if you have had a heart attack or suffer high blood pressure, cold generally, and cold water in particular, are probably best avoided. This is because the noradrenaline released under these conditions can push up the blood pressure quite severely. The rise in the amount of free-fat in the blood which follows increases the heart's oxygen consumption and the stickiness of the blood platelets, making a coronary thrombosis more likely. Such changes explain why elderly people particularly get sudden heart attacks and strokes on sudden cold immersion and when they get thoroughly chilled. An old person collapsing suddenly at a bus-stop on a cold day is a common occurrence because of these complications of getting chilled. Deaths from exposure in mountain climbers could be due either to exhaustion of their noradrenaline supplies, or to the accumulation in their blood of high concentrations of the acid breakdown products resulting from burning large amounts of fat.

For the general improvement of adult fitness, swimming in comfortably warm water would appear to be an excellent form of exercise. Again the target pulse rate zones described in the part of this chapter on gymnasium activity still apply. The amount and intensity of non-competitive swimming should be steadily stepped up to keep within these zones for ten to fifteen minute periods two or three times each week. For those already acclimatized to it, swimming in colder water outdoors may be found more invigorating than swimming indoors in comparatively warm water. This may be because it is one of turning on that drug of addiction, noradrenaline. It is also reputed to 'tone up' the skin, probably by burning off the fat and by exercising all the little muscles which pull on the hairs in the skin to give you 'goose-flesh'. In spite of these advantages I still wouldn't recommend swimming in uncomfortably cold water for the unfit.

Walking, jogging and running
Walking is one of the mildest forms of exercise you can take and given the right conditions one of the pleasantest. Unfortunately it is probably too mild to have much effect, and city streets are wet, cold or otherwise un-

pleasant. Even with unfit people walking briskly the pulse rate doesn't rise much above 100 to 110 beats per minute, way below most people's target zone for 'vigorous exercise'. This can be increased considerably by going up steep hills or flights of stairs, but the former are rare in most cities and the latter monotonous.

It remains, however, one of the best rehabilitation exercises in the first two or three months after a heart attack, forming a bridging activity leading up gradually to more vigorous exercise. It has been shown to have some long-term protective effect on reducing the number of heart attacks in people whose work involves a considerable amount of walking, such as postmen, and those who walk for at least fifteen minutes during their journey to and from work. However, these figures could of course just be another way of showing the risks of executive jobs and driving a car.

Jogging has become another very popular form of exercise for those wishing to lessen their chances of getting a heart attack, especially in America. However, there have been some instances of jogging apparently provoking heart attacks, and so this activity is at present under something of a cloud. This is a classic example of the need for care in the early stages of any exercise programme. As with the gymnasium programme those taking it up are likely to be the very people who are most at risk. In addition, a large number will be considerably overweight and will drive themselves to jog at the same pace as those who are several stone lighter. Lastly they may well start their jogging during the winter when other forms of outdoor exercise are not available, and suffer the blood pressure and fat-raising effects of cold mentioned previously.

For maximum safety and benefit therefore, would-be joggers should if necessary get their weight down by diet first and then limber up for a week or two by doing free exercises and running on the spot. Avoiding cold days, they are then ready to jog at a pace which leaves sufficient breath for carrying on a conversation.

Running suffers from similar hazards as well as

having a competitive, noradrenaline-increasing effect from casual races between the fit and unfit, old and young, lean and fat. Again, like jogging, if taken in a carefully progressive, non-competitive fashion under the right conditions, it can be an excellent form of exercise.

Football
Although in the scrum, rugby football has a more isometric, straining, pushing aspect to it than association football, it is generally played only by the relatively young and hideously fit and so is safe for the heart at least. Both games, however, have the same disadvantages from this point of view in that they are intensely competitive, involve violent bouts of erratic activity and are played often under extremely cold conditions. Also it is often when a player is most in need of keeping fit that he gives up because of age or pressure of work. Not many executives can take two afternoons off each week to play football on a ground which is usually the other side of town. Mainly this is confined to the young and fit who are least in need of the physical benefits of such recreation.

The heart and blood chemistry changes occurring during football do not appear to have been studied in the players themselves. This is a curious omission considering the enthusiasm among medical students for rugby. I hope to fill this important gap in medical knowledge in the near future. In the meantime we'll have to make do with the similar situation of professional hockey players studied in America. These showed a six-fold increase in their noradrenaline production during a game which brings them almost up to the levels reached by the racing drivers. By comparison two players who because of previous injuries were stopped by their coach from playing in the match and just had to sit on a bench and watch showed rises in adrenaline levels alone.

This brings us on to spectator sports. In this country people often consider themselves 'sportsmen' if they go to a football match, wrestling or the races, or even watch these events on television. Unfortunately it doesn't work like that. Tests have shown that when spectators at football matches get excited by the game their pulse rate often goes up to 150 beats per minute while, as would be expected, when they watch it on television it only increases to 110 beats per minute. Thus they are getting a large emotional kick out of watching but little or no physical activity to offset it and use up the extra fat and sugar released into the blood. This was dramatically demonstrated over fifty years ago by a famous American doctor called Walter B Cannon. In his book *Bodily changes in pain, hunger, fear and rage* which contains more basic truth than the majority of texts written on these subjects up to the present day, he describes finding high blood sugar levels in college students watching an important football match. This was so marked in a considerable proportion of the students that the sugar even overflowed into their urine, something which was only supposed to occur in severe diabetes! The general conclusion from this is that 'doing is better than viewing', and if you enjoy football you should join the more than one million people in this country who play it each week.

Squash and tennis
Though squash is the more intensive, these are similar sports with similar drawbacks as ways of getting and keeping fit. They are competitive and violently energetic in short bursts. It is extremely difficult to grade the severity of the exertion to suit the exact stage of fitness reached. Except in the most vigorous games of squash the pulse rate is unlikely to be kept in the optimal pulse zone for many seconds at a time, but can swing wildly above and below it according to the erratic progress of the game. Furthermore, these are relatively expensive ways for people to obtain exercise and are unlikely to fulfill the needs of the expanding population in most cities. In the case of tennis it is also a seasonal sport and cannot provide an even level of physical activity all the year round, which is what is needed for maximum benefit from the heart's point of view.

Golf

This is another exercise which almost isn't. It was once described as being just a way of spoiling a good walk. Though perhaps a rather extreme view, there could be a certain amount of truth in it. Firstly it slows the walk down to the pace of the slowest player. It can even abolish the walking element completely by introducing motorised trolleys. Secondly, it introduces a competitive element. Many people come to look on the golf course as an extension of the boardroom table, to be fought over inch by inch, tee by tee. It is also regarded as a place to meet clients and do business. Thirdly there is the infrequent violent swing, and the infuriating nature of the game itself, to add to its other blood pressure and fat-raising properties. With bunkers and rough bits in which to lose balls, and cunning slopes to take the ball away from the hole and snatch victory from your grasp, it is often more of an emotional assault course rather than a golf course.

Finally, to add to this catalogue of crimes against the good name of exercise, there are the alcoholic hazards of the nineteenth hole. Having raised your free fat levels on the other eighteen holes, the custom is to then conduct a little chemistry experiment. This involves titrating these fatty acids with a base, ethyl alcohol, to produce neutral fat, triglyceride, one of the most harmful of blood-fats. So widespread is this habit that one little girl accusingly said to her father returning late for his Sunday lunch, 'Daddy, you smell of golf!'

One of the commonest presenting symptoms of incipient coronary heart disease is the feeling of a need to take up exercise, and golf is one of the expensive activities to which the executive will naturally turn. It is therefore hardly surprising, especially in view of the above features of the sport, that the mortality rate of those who have just joined a golf club is quite high.

Other forms of exercise

As seen from the previous examples, when considering

the suitability of a particular exercise for preventing or treating heart trouble, several factors have to be taken into account. Is it mainly isometric, causing abrupt strain on the heart and blood vessels, or isotonic, evenly using and increasing their strength? Does it exercise the whole body? Can it be continued, preferably under warm conditions, all the year round? Is it easily available or prohibitively expensive? Last but not least, is it sufficiently pleasant and varied to be taken up and continued as a life-long habit by any except the most enthusiastic 'exercise nut'.

Fortunately, people vary in the type of exercise which suits them best and I apologize if your favourite sport was omitted or unfavourably reviewed in this account. Cycling to work, for instance, if it wasn't for the accident risk, would be another excellent activity. The physical action is right, particularly if there are a few moderate gradients on the way, and time may even be saved on the journey. Think of all the eccentric men and women who live to ripe old ages on bicycles. Whoever heard of a French onion salesman having a heart attack? In the Pyrenees there was alleged to be a man of seventy-five who was cited simultaneously in paternity suits by girls in five different villages roundabout, and attributed his longevity, mobility and virility to his bicycle.

On a related subject, dancing, unless taken energetically and in large amounts, appears to have little protective effect on the heart. Electro-cardiographic tracings taken this year at a British Heart Foundation dance showed that only the quick step moved the heart to beat more rapidly than 110 times a minute. It suggests that this vertical expression of a horizontal desire is insufficiently vigorous to be effective as exercise. The control needed for ballroom dancing may also introduce isometric pauses in this isotonic form of exertion.

These comments on various forms of exercise are only considered from the point of view of possible benefits to the heart and its safety. A lot of work remains to be done on studying the immediate and long term results of different sports. 'Sport for all' has become the motto of the Sports Council in this country and the finances for backing this policy with more facilities such as gymnasia, swimming pools and teachers of physical education to staff them will probably be forthcoming. To prevent unfit, middle-aged people doing themselves harm by over exertion under unsuitable conditions, perhaps 'Safe sport for all' should be the aim.

Schools have an important part to play in encouraging individual activities rather than mass spectator sports, and explaining some of the advantages of the exercise habit. Above all, they should try not to put people off exercise for life by over-emphasis on its competitive side. Many large business firms and other organizations could set an example in this direction and prolong the lives of their staff by concentrating less on large sports-grounds miles away, and much more on the on-the-spot facilities which I have described. These could be used by people throughout the day, all the year round, and become an integral part of their daily lives to the benefit of employer and employee alike.

8. The message

There is a great deal of lip-service at present being paid to the idea of preventing pollution of the external environment, though there appears to be little that the average mortal can do to deflect the avalanche of industrial wastes, disposable containers and surplus people threatening to engulf him. The object of this book is to describe some ways in which pollution of the internal environment can occur by the over-production of acid wastes in response to the aggressive emotions induced by the modern pattern of living.

There are many parallels between pollution of the external and internal environments. Not only does the former process directly contribute to the latter, but the form of blood vessel degeneration causing heart attacks can be thought of as being due to excess oil, which is what fat is at body temperature, washed up onto the arterial beaches. An example of many of the factors involved in this process is one of the most popular fictional heroes of the Western world, James Bond. His fabled existence, as retailed in the highly successful books and multi-million-pound films made from them, shows in an exaggerated form the patterns of behaviour which enables this *alter ego* to destroy his creator. Even in early childhood, Ian Fleming was all set for a coronary career of the 'Mr West' type described earlier. From being a large, healthy, exceedingly naughty child, 'the difficult one' of the family as John Pearson describes him in his biography, he went on to become a *Victor Ludorum* at Eton two years in succession. He was particularly outstanding in the gruelling long-distance athletic events, showing extreme style, strength and will-power. This, as he later himself admitted, was achieved largely because of his role of second son trying to compensate for a brilliant elder brother.

In the process it seems likely that he learned the knack of turning on large supplies of the self-administered drug, noradrenaline. Recent tests on athletes suggest that this hormone could be the biochemical basis of willpower. Top class athletes were found to have very high levels of this hormone in their blood at the end of races. Because of its ability to override stress symptoms, it may enable them to raise their pain threshold for the duration of the event. They can then tolerate the very high concentration of lactic acid that accumulates in muscles during maximum effort and would otherwise prevent further exertion. It may provide a biochemical explanation of why the best athletes, especially when spurred on by the cheering of their supporters and the element of competition in a close race, can drive themselves through the pain barrier.

This habit, and the feeling of almost superhuman power and strength which arises from it, once experienced is never forgotten. It is then brought into play whenever possible, especially at times of physical and mental crises, giving great stamina and resilience, but at a cost.

Ian Fleming led a strenuous early life. After some initial skirmishes with Sandhurst and the Foreign Office, he entered journalism and then stockbroking. War came as something of a relief from routine, and he had a chequered career in Naval Intelligence which gave him the factual material on weaponry and commando tactics used in the books, which he suddenly started writing at the age of forty-three.

Five years earlier he had the first warning symptoms of heart disease. He was then smoking over sixty cigarettes and drinking more than a quarter-bottle of gin every day. Despite the advice offered by the best heart specialists in England and America, he continued to smoke his 300 hand-made Morland cigarettes each week, and often double this number. This obsession with cigarettes was incorporated, as with his materialism, his drinking and casual use of women, in what has been described as his 'undercover autobiography', the Bond books. In many ways it must have been a relief for Fleming to exteriorise these thoughts, a type of profitable abreactive psychotherapy. Some of the pent-up emotion gushes out in a revealing fashion in the first paragraph of his first book, *Casino Royale*:

> The scent and smoke and sweat of a casino are nauseating at three in the morning. Then the soul-erosion produced by high gambling – compost of greed and fear and nervous tension – becomes unbearable and the senses awake and revolt from it.

He is, I suggest, unconsciously describing the same mixture of emotion which erodes the heart.

As Bond flourished over the next twelve years, so Fleming's health and spirits waned. It was as though his brain-child had become almost a cancerous growth, feeding on the restless energy bottled up inside him. While Bond was on the loose 'kiss-kissing', 'bang-banging' his way through continents and people, his creator was left with one divorce, several law-suits, and a steadily worsening heart. His standard reaction to all advice from physicians is best summed up under the title *Dr No*.

His reasons for this determined course of self-destruction are those of most noradrenaline addicts, that only when he could unlock his supplies of this vital drug, whether by cigarettes or re-living the thrills enjoyed by his fantasy character, did he feel truly alive. He finally put his own epitaph under James Bond's name. It read 'I shall not waste my days in trying to prolong them. I shall use my time.'

Doctors must, and most of us coronary candidates will, agree with this philosophy of not striving officiously to keep alive and yet would like to remain well enough to both use and enjoy a full span of life. The title of Ian Fleming's last book *You only live twice* suggests a compromise solution. That is that your first life is till the age of forty, or your first coronary, which ever comes sooner. Till then you live whatever variety of the Western way of life you choose, wining, dining and womanizing to taste, keeping only to the limits dictated by conscience, society and career.

The first coronary attack, which an increasing number of men are managing to achieve in their thirties by strict devotion to excesses in all parts of their first life, can be considered a dress rehearsal of death. Thanks to improvements in caring for the acute coronary case, only thirty per cent die of their first heart attack, and the rest are let off with a caution. However, this is the clearest sign that the writing is on the walls of their blood vessels for those who care to read it. This is the time they need to make a choice of whether they sincerely want to live their second life or not. Ian Fleming had become disillusioned and apparently decided against it. This is a pity because the second life, beginning, as the saying goes, 'at forty', would seem to have a great deal to offer. The worst of the insecurities and uncertainties of youth are over and you have with luck found the things that you enjoy and are best at doing, as well as learning to avoid some of the situations you find most unpleasant. You have made, or are well on the way to making, whatever money or position for which you can hope. By getting your 'second wind' it should be possible to make a prolonged plateau of your success rather than a briefly enjoyed pinnacle.

Preparation for the second life needs an education process just as much as the first. Some will have gained sufficient insight to educate themselves but others need help. Many physicians see a heart attack as an illness which happens by chance, to be treated in hospital, and then ignored in the hope that it will go away and never come back. This is rather like dragging a drowning man onto a raft, giving him artificial respiration and then throwing him back into the sea to sink or swim as best he can.

What is needed is a 'Second Life School' to which those who would like help with balancing the accounts at the end of their first life, and shaping up to the second, could go. This team of advisers would be led by a 'mediatrician', a doctor specializing in the problems of the middle-aged, just as the pediatrician looks after the young and the geriatrician the elderly. He would be helped in this renaissance activity by both physio- and psychothera-pists. Such a team could also help people choose from a wide range of extended adult education programmes to catch up on things they feel they missed the first time round, or even to choose a new career if they want a change of occupation. Women might welcome the oppor-tunity to take up new careers or interests in their second life outside the home.

A physical and emotional audit would be the first essential at the start of the second life and most people would start off with an overdraft which was proportional to how much they had failed to balance these factors in their first life. Charles Colton summed it up over 150 years ago when he wrote: 'The excesses of our youth are drafts upon our old age, payable with interest, about twenty years after date.' A general medical examination including heart and blood chemistry checks with special emphasis on blood fats would give a good idea of your condition at the start of the second life. A range of options for maintaining and improving health could then be offered and the checks repeated at intervals so that each person can see for themselves how changes in their pattern of living affect their bodies. Such a 'bio-feedback' system is built into the idea of regular exercise, since a reduction in the exertion which is possible without strain becomes obvious whenever people get emotionally over-loaded at work or at home.

These ideas make no claim to originality, but are re-statements of self-evident truths which are ignored, or at least certainly not acted upon in Western societies today. It is an interesting paradox that having set out to study what appeared to be a modern malaise by the most up-to-date scientific methods, the trail leads back to antiquity, where the causes and remedies were well recognized from practical experience. Atheromatous arterial degeneration has been found in Egyptian mummies, so it is not a new disease. In the Old Testament it is also stated that 'envy and wrath shorten life'.

Much of the latest research work in this book is taken up with showing the biochemical effects of what used to be looked on as 'sinning'. The results suggest that in modern society wrath, reinforced by sloth and gluttony, is the deadliest of the seven sins. Some people find a religious answer to this problem. In fact it was demon-strated in a big study in Framingham, Massachusetts that people who went regularly to church suffered half as many heart attacks as those in the same community who didn't. Others would say that the seven sins are like exam questions, not more than three of which should be attempted at one time.

Sloth is particularly deadly, and the use of physical activity as a natural antidote to emotional stress was clearly recognized and stated by Plato as already mentioned in connection with the great benefits of regular vigorous exercise. Aristotle, too, heralded the theory of disturbed hormonal balance with his sug-gestion that imbalance between the four 'humours' caused disease. Again recent research has shown how 'choler' can raise 'cholesterol' and lead on to cardiac illness.

In ancient India, as early as 300 BC, the dangers of excessive materialism were recognized. The Brahmin way of life shows how affluence can be used to advantage by dividing a man's life into four stages, those of study, achievement, disengagement and ultimate contentment.

129

This is similar to the idea of living twice suggested here, and may indicate an Eastern solution to a Western problem.

Though there were probably other examples of similar ideas recurring at an earlier date, the idea of two lives appears again in the writings of Lewis Cornaro, a venerable Venetian gentleman who died in 1566 aged over a hundred years. Apart from his name being an almost exact anagram of coronary, he has the distinction that his collected works written at the ages of eighty-three, eighty-six and ninety-one, were a sufficiently good argument for his ideas to be translated from the Italian and re-published in 1825. In his collected works entitled *Sure methods of attaining a long and healthfull life,* he states that the safest way is 'at least after forty to embrace sobriety. This is no such difficult affair since we are all human beings and endowed with reason, consequently we are master of all our actions. This sobriety is reduced to two things, quality and quantity. The first, namely quality, consists in nothing but not eating food or drinking wines prejudicial to the stomach. The second, which is quantity, consists in not eating or drinking more than the stomach can easily digest, which quantity and quality every man should be a perfect judge of by the time he is forty, or fifty or sixty, and whoever observes these two rules may be said to live a regular and sober life. This is of so much virtue and efficacy that the humours of such a man's body become most homogeneous, harmonious and perfect; and when thus improved are no longer liable to be corrupted or disturbed by any other disorders whatsoever, such as suffering excessive heat or cold, too much fatigue, want of natural rest, and the like, unless of the last degree of excess. Wherefore since the humours of persons, who observe these two rules relative to eating and drinking cannot possibly be corrupted and engender acute diseases, the sources of untimely death, every man is bound to comply with them; for whoever acts otherwise, living a disorderly instead of a regular life, is constantly exposed to disease and mortality.'

Substitute the word 'biochemistry' for 'humours', and

it is difficult to improve on two of the basic recommendations for the second life!

The other agents which can be employed at this time according to taste and need are equally well summed up in the 1825 introductions to the writings of Cornaro: 'It is a kind of regimen into which every man may put himself without interruption to business, expense of money or loss of time. If exercise throws off all superfluities, temperance prevents them; if exercise clears the vessels, temperance neither satiates nor overstrains them; if exercise raises proper ferments in the humours and promotes the circulation of the blood, temperance gives nature her full play and enables her to exert herself in all her force and vigour; if exercise dissipates a growing distemper, temperance starves it.

'Physic for the most part is nothing else but the substitute of exercise or temperance. Medicines are indeed absolutely necessary in acute distempers, that cannot wait the slow operations of these two great instruments of health; but, were man to live in an habitual course of exercise and temperance, there would be but little occasion for them. Accordingly we find that those parts of the world are most healthy, where they subsist by the chase, and that men live longest when their lives were employed in hunting and when they had little food besides what they caught. Blistering, cupping and bleeding are seldom of use, but to the idle and intemperate, as all those inward applications, which are so much in practice among us, are for the most part nothing else but expedients to make luxury consistent with health. The apothecary is perpetually employed in undermining the cook and the vintner.'

Substituting heart transplants and vein grafts for the earlier surgical remedies mentioned and the range of options and their relative merit remain the same today. Patients awaiting trial by cardiac surgery frequently find that if their preparation for the event includes a strict reducing diet and carefully regulated exercise, by the time they are ready for surgery they are ready to do without it.

Conversely, it is found that putting new arteries or even complete hearts into patients who make no other change to their way of life often results in rapidly occurring thrombosis of their new blood vessels. The life-style for the second life needs to be determined by any residual physical disability from the first intensity of current emotional stress and by personal choice in achieving a balance between the amount eaten and the amount used up by exercise. This calorie balance can be achieved by eating and drinking reasonably liberally and exercising vigorously and often. The alternative is to reduce intake and hence the amount of exercise needed to offset it, though a moderate level of exertion is still advisable to balance an emotionally active life. With these provisos and, where necessary, a firm resolve to drive less, smoke less and delegate more, it should be possible to have a long, healthy and enjoyable life.

These ideas are directed to anyone who finds the arguments put forward reasonable and relevant to their style of living. They cannot be imposed by doctor or spouse as they rely on actions taken from insight. They attempt to apply some of the knowledge gained during 4,000 years of civilization to a disease of civilized man. Though the serious subject of heart disease is tackled from many irreverent angles in this book, it is only in an attempt to stimulate thought, discussion and whenever possible action, on the underlying ideas. I have lost too many teachers, friends and relatives from this modern epidemic to have anything other than a healthy respect for the complex network of factors underlying this disease. The message remains that the Western way of life is the main cause of what has become the Western way of death.

Appendix

Literature

Although some of the views expressed in *The Western Way of Death* are personal and subject to controversy, I have tried to maintain a substratum of fact. The main sources of both the facts and theories discussed in this book are listed here according to chapter, the detailed references being given in the bibliography.

Chapter 1

History of heart disease: Guthrie, 1945; Ruffer, 1911; Wellcome Institute of the History of Medicine Catalogue, 1970; Harvey, 1628.

Emotion and the heart: Osler, 1910; Cannon, 1929; Friedman and Rosenman, 1957, 1959; Rosenman *et al.*, 1964, 1966, 1970; Carruthers, 1969; Morris, 1967.

Chapter 2

Urban pressures: Morris, 1969; Levi, 1971; Carlestam and Levi, 1971, Packer, 1974.

Chapter 3
Motor racing: Taggart *et al.*, 1969; Taggart and Carruthers, 1971, 1972.
Traffic driving: Taggart and Gibbons, 1967; Bellet *et al.*, 1969.

Chapter 4
Accountants: Friedman and Rosenman, 1959; Rosenman *et al.*, 1966, 1970
Clerical workers: Levi, 1971.
Industrial stress: Levi, 1972.
Bus drivers: Morris *et al.*, 1966.
Pilots: Euler and Lundberg, 1954; Carruthers, 1973.
Public speakers and television performers: Somerville *et al.*, 1971; Taggart *et al.*, 1973.

Chapter 5
Social stress and illness: Rahe *et al.*, 1964; Holmes and Rahe, 1967.
The coronary characters: Nixon, 1972; Schneider, 1956, 1967.
Television and film watching: Levi, 1972; Carruthers and Taggart, 1973.

Chapter 6
Food and drink: Carruthers, G. B., 1962.
Aspirin: Wood, 1972.
Beta-blocking drugs: Carruthers *et al.*, 1973.
Cigarettes: Murchison and Fife, 1966; Russel, 1971.
Clofibrate: Oliver *et al.*, 1972.
Coffee and tea: Yudkin, 1964; Boston Collaborative Drug Surveillance Program, 1972.
Diet: Oliver and Boyd 1961; Miettinen, 1972.

Chapter 7
The 'Bond' image: Pearson, 1966.
Living twice: Fleming, 1964; Cornaro, 1530; Hawley, 1967.

Bibliography

Bellet, S., Roman, L., and Kostis, J., *The effects of automobile driving on catecholamine and adrenocortical excretion.* American Journal of Cardiology, 24, 365, 1969

Boston Collaborative Drug Surveillance Program, *Coffee drinking and acute myocardial infarction.* Lancet, 2, 1278, 1972

Cannon, W. B., *Bodily changes in pain, hunger, fear and rage.* D. Appleton, New York, 1929

Carlestam, G. and Levi, L., *Urban conglomerates as phychosocial human stressors.* Ministry of Foreign Affairs, Sweden, 1971

Carruthers, G. B., *How to live with your heart.* Evans Brothers Ltd, London, 1962

Carruthers, M. E., *Aggression and atheroma.* Lancet, 1, 1170, 1969

Carruthers, M. E., *Maintaining the cardiovascular fitness of pilots.* Lancet, 1, 1048, 1973

135

Carruthers, M. E. and Taggart, P., *The vagotonicity of violence*. British Medical Journal, 3, 384, 1973

Carruthers, M. E., Taggart, P. and Somerville, W., *Some effects of β-blockade on the lipid response to certain emotions*. Ciba Symposium 'New Perspectives in B-blockade' proceedings, 1973

Cornaro, L., *Sure methods of attaining a long and healthfull life*. 1530, republished in 1825.

Euler, U. S. von, and Lundberg, U., *Effects of flying on the epinephrine excretion in Air Force personnel*. Journal of Applied Physiology, 6, 551, 1954

Fleming, I., *You only live twice*. Jonathan Cape, London, 1964

Friedman, M. and Rosenman, R. H., *Comparison of fat intake of American men and women*. Circulation, 16, 339, 1957

Friedman, M. and Rosenman, R. H., *Association of pecific overt behaviour pattern with blood and cardiovascular findings*. Journal of the American Medical Association, 169, 1268, 1959

Guthrie, D., *A history of medicine*. Thomas Nelson, London, 1945

Harvey, W., *The circulation of the blood* (1628). Everyman's Library, 1907.

Hawley, C., *The Hurricane Years*. 1967

Holmes, T. H. and Rahe, R. H., *The social readjustment rating scale*. Journal of Psychosomatic Research, 2, 213, 1967

Levi, L., *Emotional Stress*. Karger, New York, 1967

Levi, L., Editor *Society, Stress and Disease*, Volume 1, *The psychosocial environment and psychosomatic disease*. Oxford University Press, 1971

Levi, L., *Stress and distress*. Oxford University Press, 1971

Miettinen, M. et al. *Effect of cholesterol lowering diet on mortality from coronary heart disease and other causes*. Lancet, 2, 835, 1972

Morris, D., *The Naked Ape*. Jonathan Cape, London, 1967

Morris, D., *The Human Zoo.* Jonathan Cape, London, 1969

Morris, J. N., et al, *Incidence and prediction of ischaemic heart disease in London Busmen.* Lancet, 2, 553, 1966

Morris, J. N. *et al., Vigorous exercise in leisure time and the incidence of coronary heart-disease.* Lancet, 1, 333, 1973

Murchison, L. E. and Fyfe, T., *Effects of cigarette smoking on serum lipids, blood-glucose, and platelet adhesiveness.* Lancet, 1, 182, 1966

Nixon, P., *Recovery from coronary illness.* Rehabilitation, 81, 23, 1972

Nixon, P., and Carruthers, M. E., *A British pilot study of exercise therapy, II. The cardiac patient.* British Medical *Journal,* 1974 in press

Oliver, M. F., and Boyd, G. S., *Influence of reduction of serum lipids in prognosis of coronary heart disease.* Lancet, 2, 499, 1961

Oliver, M. F. *et al., The Edinburgh trial of Clofibrate,* British Medical Journal, 3, 912, 1972

Osler, W., *Angina pectoris,* Lancet, 1, 839, 1910

Packer, E., *Stress in your life,* Orbis Publishing, 1974

Plato (380 BC), *Timaeus and Critias* (translated by D. Lee). Penguin Books, 1971

Raab, W., *Preventive myocardiology – proposals for social action,* in 'Society, Stress and Disease', editor L. Levi, Oxford University Press, 1971

Rahe, R. H. *et al., Social stress and illness onset.* Journal of Psychosomatic Research, 8, 35, 1964

Rosenman, R. H., *et al., A predictive study of coronary heart disease. The Western Collaborative Group Study.* Journal of the American Medical Association, 189, 15, 1964

Rosenman, R. H. *et al., Western Collaborative Group Study: A follow-up experience of two years.* Journal of the American Medical Association, 195, 86, 1966

Rosenham, R. H. *et al., Coronary heart disease in the Western Collaborative Group Study. A follow-up experience of $4\frac{1}{2}$ years.* Journal of Chronic Diseases, 23, 173, 1970

Ruffer, M.A., *On arterial lesions found in Egyptian mummies.* Journal of Pathology and Bacteriology, 15, 453, 1911

Russel, M. A. H., *Cigarette dependence: 1 – Nature and classification. II – Doctor's role in management.* British Medical Journal, 2, 330, 1971

Schneider, D. E., *The image of the heart.* International University Press Inc., New York, 1956

Schneider, D. E., *Psychoanalysis of heart attack.* Dial Press Inc., New York, 1967

Somerville, W., Taggart, P., and Carruthers, M. E. (1972). *Cardiovascular responses to public speaking and their modification by oxprenolol.* CIBA symposium, 'New perspectives in β-blockade', proceedings, 1973

Taggart, P., and Gibbons, D., *Motor-car driving and the heart rate.* British Medical Journal, 1, 411, 1967

Taggart, P., and Carruthers, M. E., *Endogenous hyperlipidaemia induced by the emotional stress of racing driving.* Lancet, 1, 363, 1971

Taggart, P., and Carruthers, M. E., *Suppression by oxprenolol of adrenergic response to stress.* Lancet, 2, 256, 1972

Taggart, P., Gibbons, D., and Somerville, W., *Some effects of motor-car driving on the normal and abnormal heart.* British Medical Journal, 4, 130, 1969

Taggart, P., Carruthers, M. E. and Somerville, W., *Speaking before an audience: Observations on the electrocardiagram, plasma catecholamines and lipids, and their modification by oxprenolol.* Lancet 2, 341, 1973

Wellcome Institute of the History of Medicine Exhibition Catalogue, 1970. *The History of Cardiology*

Wood, L., *Aspirin and myocardial infarction.* Lancet, 2, 1021, 1972

Yudkin, J., *Levels of dietary sucrose in patients with occlusive atherosclerotic disease.* Lancet, 2, 4, 1964

Index

Index

Index

About the Author

Dr Malcolm Carruthers, MD, MRCPath, was born in London in 1938 and educated at Highgate School and the Middlesex Hospital. From 1961 to 1970 he was in general practice in Highgate, although for the last five years of this period he was also training in Pathology at the Middlesex Hospital. Leaving general practice, he was appointed Senior Lecturer in Chemical Pathology at the Institute of Ophthalmology, and in 1972 he left to take up his post as Senior Lecturer in the Research Chemical Pathology Department at St Mary's Hospital Medical School.

Dr Carruthers has carried out a great deal of original research into both the emotional and physical aspects of the stress which causes heart disease.